CW01433606

SEASONAL AFFECTIVE DISORDER

UNDERSTANDING SAD, HOLISTIC TREATMENTS FOR
LASTING SOLUTIONS: RESOURCE GUIDE FOR PEOPLE
AFFECTED BY SAD

L. A. LEES BSN CHPN

© **Copyright L.A. Lees BSN CHPN 2024 - All rights reserved.**

The content within this book may not be reproduced, duplicated or transmitted without direct written permission from the author or the publisher.

Under no circumstances will any blame or legal responsibility be held against the publisher, or author, for any damages, reparation, or monetary loss due to the information contained within this book. Either directly or indirectly. You are responsible for your own choices, actions, and results.

Legal Notice:

This book is copyright protected. This book is only for personal use. You cannot amend, distribute, sell, use, quote or paraphrase any part, of the content within this book, without the consent of the author or publisher.

Disclaimer Notice:

Please note the information contained within this document is for educational and entertainment purposes only. All effort has been expended to present accurate, up-to-date, and reliable, complete information. No warranties of any kind are declared or implied. Readers acknowledge that the author is not engaging in the rendering of legal, financial, medical or professional advice. The content within this book has been derived from various sources. Please consult a licensed professional before attempting any techniques outlined in this book.

By reading this document, the reader agrees that under no circumstances is the author responsible for any losses, direct or indirect, which are incurred as a result of the use of the information contained within this document, including, but not limited to, — errors, omissions, or inaccuracies.

Written with love to honor my sister Dana, and all those who are affected by SAD

TABLE OF CONTENTS

INTRODUCTION

Every winter, as the days shorten and the darkness swells, millions find themselves grappling with the weight of diminished sunlight. Seasonal Affective Disorder (SAD), a condition often cloaked in the guise of mere "winter blues," is far more pervasive and debilitating than many realize. Consider the stark reality: up to 10% of the population in northern latitudes suffers from SAD, experiencing symptoms that can severely disrupt their daily lives.

As someone who has navigated the icy waters of SAD alongside family, friends, and patients, I've witnessed firsthand the profound impact it can have—not just on those directly afflicted, but on the people close to them as well. My journey through understanding and managing this condition has not only deepened my empathy but has equipped me with insights that I am eager to share with you. This book is a culmination of years of learning, both professional and personal, distilled into guidance that, I hope, will illuminate your path as much as it did mine.

The purpose of this book is clear: to furnish you with a thorough understanding of Seasonal Affective Disorder. By integrating scientific research with real-life stories, I aim to arm you with knowledge and strategies to effectively manage SAD. From identifying symptoms to exploring comprehensive treatment options and coping mechanisms, this guide seeks to empower you and your loved ones to reclaim joy and balance throughout the seasons.

This resource is crafted for adults experiencing SAD, as well as their family and friends who are committed to supporting them. Recognizing the unique challenges faced by each individual, this book strives to be a versatile tool—informative yet easy to navigate, enriched with expert advice yet relatable through personal anecdotes.

Structured to foster clarity and ease of understanding, the book unfolds across several key sections. We begin by exploring the nature of SAD, its symptoms, and triggers. Subsequent chapters delve into effective treatment modalities, from light therapy and medication to lifestyle adjustments and psychological therapies. We also dedicate special attention to how supporters can aid those struggling with SAD, ensuring that no one has to walk this path alone. Lastly, we'll tackle some nuanced topics for those looking for an in-depth understanding.

What sets this book apart is its holistic approach. It is not merely an academic overview but a practical companion filled with the latest findings and heartfelt stories from individuals who have lived through the lows and highs of SAD. By providing actionable advice, I hope to transform knowledge into power—the power for you to navigate SAD with confidence and optimism.

In closing, let this book serve as a beacon of hope. Seasonal Affective Disorder, while challenging, does not define you or dictate the quality of your life. With the right tools and understanding, you can adjust the sails on your journey through the colder months and emerge resilient. Let's step forward together, equipped to face SAD with renewed strength and assurance.

I invite you now to turn the page, engage with this material, and apply it meaningfully to your life or supporting someone you care about. Together, we can face the winter's challenge and move toward a brighter, more balanced tomorrow.

1

THE BASICS OF SAD

A s the leaves begin to change color and a chill permeates the air, many anticipate the cozy comforts of autumn and the jovial festivities of winter. However, for a significant portion of the population, these seasonal shifts herald a much darker time. Seasonal Affective Disorder (SAD), a type of depression that occurs at a specific time of year, typically in the fall and winter months, although there are less common forms of SAD in other months. It is more than just a trivial case of the "winter blues." It is a recognized medical condition that can profoundly affect every aspect of a person's life, from their energy levels and appetite to their sleep patterns, ability to enjoy life's moments, and much more.

Understanding SAD in its full complexity is paramount not only for those directly experiencing its effects, but also for their families, friends, and colleagues who might struggle to comprehend the changes seen in their loved ones. This chapter aims to peel back the layers of SAD, debunking common myths and providing a clear picture of its symptoms, diagnosis, and societal perceptions.

By fostering a more in-depth understanding of SAD, we can begin to dismantle the stigma associated with this condition and pave the way for better support systems and treatments.

1.1 DECODING SAD: SYMPTOMS, DIAGNOSIS, AND MISCONCEPTIONS

Understanding Symptoms

Seasonal Affective Disorder manifests in a variety of symptoms that may initially be dismissed as mere signs of winter lethargy. However, the impact of SAD is far-reaching, affecting emotional and physical health in several ways. Emotionally, individuals may experience persistent sadness, anxiety, a sense of hopelessness, and even feelings of guilt or worthlessness. These symptoms are often accompanied by a loss of interest in activities once enjoyed, leading to social withdrawal and isolation. Physically, SAD can present as significant changes in sleep patterns—whether it's insomnia or oversleeping—appetite changes, particularly an increased craving for carbohydrates, and notable weight gain. Additionally, many report feeling lethargic, experiencing a significant decrease in energy levels, or finding it difficult to concentrate.

The cyclical pattern of these symptoms is what often sets SAD apart from other forms of depression. They typically begin in the fall, as daylight decreases, and not only persist, but often times worsen through the winter months, then resolve during spring and summer. Recognizing this pattern is key in diagnosing SAD and distinguishing it from other psychiatric conditions, which brings us to the definitive process of diagnosis.

Navigating Diagnosis

Diagnosing SAD involves a careful evaluation by healthcare professionals, who must rule out other potential causes of depression. The diagnostic process typically includes a thorough review of the individual's medical history, a physical examination, and detailed discussions about mood and behavior patterns. Clinicians use specific diagnostic criteria from the Diagnostic and Statistical Manual of Mental Disorders (DSM-5) to ensure accuracy. These criteria emphasize the seasonal pattern of major depressive episodes occurring during specific times of the year, resolving at others, and happening consecutively for at least two years. One of the most significant challenges in diagnosing SAD is ensuring that it is not confused with other types of depressive disorders. This is definitive as the treatment for SAD, including light therapy, antidepressants, and cognitive-behavioral therapy, may differ from other depressions. Accurate diagnosis is therefore pivotal to effective management, emphasizing the need for heightened awareness and understanding of this disorder among both the public and medical professionals.

Addressing Misconceptions

Despite its prevalence and impact, numerous misconceptions about SAD persist, which can hinder effective treatment and support. One common myth is that SAD is merely a minor inconvenience—a trivial dislike of winter or bad weather. This misconception minimizes the true difficulty faced by those affected and can prevent them from seeking necessary treatment. Another widespread falsehood is the belief that SAD can be overcome through sheer willpower, or that it is a sign of personal weakness. Such stigmas can lead to significant guilt and reluctance to discuss symptoms or pursue help.

It is vital to challenge these misconceptions and spread accurate information to foster a more empathetic and supportive environment. Understanding SAD as a legitimate medical condition with a biological basis can encourage affected individuals and their support networks to take the symptoms seriously and seek appropriate treatment.

Public Perception

The way SAD is viewed by society has profound implications for those who suffer from it. Despite growing awareness, there remains a significant lack of understanding about SAD, often leading to stigma and social isolation for those affected. The trivialization of SAD as just "winter blues" overlooks the severity of the disorder and can prevent individuals from acknowledging their condition and seeking help.

Efforts to educate the public about SAD must be intensified. Increased awareness can lead to greater empathy and support, encouraging those affected to come forward and access the care they need. Public health campaigns, media coverage, education programs, and books such as this one, can play crucial roles in changing perceptions and providing accurate information about SAD's symptoms, treatments, and coping strategies.

By addressing these key areas in understanding SAD—its symptoms, the process of diagnosis, the misconceptions surrounding it, and public perception—we can begin to dismantle the barriers to effective care and support. As we move forward to explore the scientific underpinnings and treatment options for SAD in the following sections, keep in mind the importance of a supportive and informed community in managing this challenging condition.

1.2 THE SCIENCE OF LIGHT AND DARKNESS ON HUMAN MOOD

The intricate dance between light and darkness plays a fundamental role in regulating human mood and behavior, a dynamic deeply intertwined with the mechanics of our biological clocks, or circadian rhythms. These internal clocks are finely tuned systems orchestrated by the brain, responding primarily to light signals to help prepare our bodies for what we naturally expect to be periods of wakefulness or sleep. As daylight wanes in the late autumn and winter months, the disruption to this light-dark cycle can profoundly impact our circadian rhythms, leading to significant mood alterations characteristic of Seasonal Affective Disorder.

Circadian rhythms dictate not just sleep patterns but also fluctuate throughout the day to influence hormone release, eating habits, digestion, and body temperature. When these rhythms go awry, as often seen in SAD, individuals might experience a range of symptoms from sleep disturbances to depression. The reduced level of sunlight in fall and winter may cause the brain to produce higher levels of melatonin, a hormone that regulates sleep, leading to increased sleepiness and a sluggish feel. Conversely, the darker days may reduce the production of serotonin, a neurotransmitter that influences mood, appetite, and sleep, often dubbed the 'feel-good' hormone. The imbalance of these hormones can precipitate the mood dips and fatigue commonly associated with SAD.

Diving deeper into the hormonal interplay, it's essential to understand how melatonin and serotonin orchestrate a delicate balance that affects our well-being. Serotonin levels are boosted by sunlight, which explains why our mood might elevate on bright sunny days. Conversely, darkness triggers the release of melatonin, preparing the body for sleep. In the winter months, the extended periods of darkness can lead to an overproduction of melatonin, making individuals feel sleepier and lethargic. At the same time, the lack of sunlight causes a drop in serotonin levels, potentially leading to depression. For those suffering from SAD, this hormonal imbalance is at the heart of many symptomatic expressions of the disorder.

Moreover, sunlight plays a critical role in the synthesis of vitamin D, a nutrient intricately linked to mood regulation. Vitamin D receptors are found widely throughout the brain, including areas linked to the development of depression. Some studies suggest that a lack of sufficient vitamin D during the darker months could lead to decreased serotonin levels, further contributing to the depressive states seen in SAD. This vitamin is not only essential for bone health but also for optimal brain function, influencing the production of neurotransmitters like serotonin and dopamine, which affect how we feel.

Given the significant impact of light on our biological rhythms and mood, light therapy emerges as a foundational treatment for SAD. This therapy involves exposure to a bright light that mimics natural sunlight, administered through a variety of devices. One basic device is known as a light box, which emits far more lumens than a customary household light. The principle behind light therapy is straightforward yet effective: by simulating the sunrise, light therapy can reset the internal biological clock, reduce excess melatonin production, and increase serotonin levels, thereby alleviating the symptoms of SAD. Typically, light therapy is recommended for about 20 to 30 minutes each morning throughout the winter months, offering a beacon of relief for those grappling with seasonal depression. This treatment aligns closely with our understanding of how light influences our circadian rhythms and hormonal balances, providing a controlled environment to reintroduce the equilibrium disrupted by the seasonal shift in natural light exposure.

As we continue to explore the complexities of Seasonal Affective Disorder, the interplay of light, biological rhythms, and hormonal balances remains a central theme. Understanding these relationships not only sheds light on why certain individuals may be more susceptible to SAD but also guides us in optimizing treatment approaches that address these fundamental disruptions. The journey through understanding SAD is as much about recognizing the biological underpinnings of our mood fluctuations as it is about finding effective interventions to mitigate these changes.

1.3 SAD VS. WINTER BLUES: KNOWING THE DIFFERENCE

Understanding the distinction between Seasonal Affective Disorder (SAD) and the more commonly experienced winter blues is important for both effective treatment and the broader recognition of SAD as a serious mental health issue. While both conditions share certain superficial similarities—occurring primarily during the colder, darker months and manifesting as mood disturbances—their similarities largely end there. Seasonal Affective Disorder is a clinically recognized form of depression that significantly impairs an individual's functioning, both socially and professionally, whereas the winter blues, or sub-syndromal SAD, generally refers to a milder, more manageable feeling of sadness or melancholy associated with winter's reduced daylight hours.

The differences in symptom severity between SAD and winter blues are stark and serve as a primary method for differential diagnosis. Those suffering from SAD often experience profound disruptions to their daily life. This could manifest as a pervasive sense of despair, loss of interest in nearly all activities, significant weight changes, and even thoughts of self-harm or suicide. In contrast, individuals experiencing the winter blues typically report feeling slightly more lethargic than usual or mildly down, but they retain the ability to find pleasure in activities and maintain their routine lifestyle. For example, while someone with the winter blues may hesitate to go out on a particularly dark, cold evening, another with SAD might find it nearly impossible to muster the energy to get out of bed for days or weeks at a time.

The necessity of distinguishing between these two conditions cannot be overstated, primarily because it influences the treatment approach. SAD, given its severity and potential implications on one's health and well-being, often requires a multifaceted treatment strategy that may include light therapy, psychotherapy, and medication. On the other hand, the winter blues might be relieved by simpler measures such as increasing exposure to natural light, exercising, and maintaining a balanced diet. Misdiagnosis or the dismissal of SAD as mere winter blues can lead to inadequate treatment, leaving the individual vulnerable to worsening symptoms and the associated risks.

Moreover, raising awareness about these distinctions is necessary in changing public perceptions and ensuring those affected receive appropriate support. Despite increasing visibility, there remains a significant portion of the population that either remains unaware of SAD or fails to grasp its seriousness, often equating it with the winter blues and thus minimizing the experiences of those truly affected by the disorder. This lack of awareness can extend to healthcare providers as well, potentially leading to underdiagnoses or misdiagnosis, thereby denying individuals the treatments that could substantially alleviate their suffering.

Educational initiatives and awareness campaigns are essential in bridging this knowledge gap. They can provide clear, accessible information that helps the public and healthcare professionals alike understand the nuances between these conditions. For instance, highlighting key symptoms exclusive to SAD in public health messages or offering screening tools that help distinguish it from less severe mood disturbances can play a significant role in improving diagnosis accuracy. Moreover, such efforts can foster a more empathetic and supportive environment, encouraging individuals experiencing any form of seasonal mood disturbances to seek help without fear of stigma or dismissal.

As we move forward in our exploration of SAD, it's important to keep these distinctions in mind, ensuring that our discussions about treatment and support are informed by a clear understanding of the condition's specific characteristics. This knowledge not only aids in crafting more effective management strategies, but also in advocating for those who endure the profound impact of Seasonal Affective Disorder.

1.4 THE IMPACT OF SAD ON DAILY LIFE AND RELATIONSHIPS

Seasonal Affective Disorder, while primarily a personal health concern, casts a wide net that can ensnare every aspect of one's social and professional life. The insidious nature of its symptoms often leads to a gradual withdrawal from social activities—a retreat that might initially be as imperceptible as the shortening days of autumn but becomes starkly apparent as the full brunt of the disorder takes hold. This withdrawal is not born out of a disinterest in social engagements but rather from the overwhelming fatigue and sadness that hallmark SAD. The energy required to simply get through the day leaves little to spare for dinners with friends or family gatherings, which, though joyful occasions, can feel like monumental tasks to someone grappling with depression. Furthermore, the irritability and hypersensitivity to rejection that often accompany SAD can strain relationships, leading to misunderstandings and conflict. The result is a vicious cycle where social isolation deepens the depressive symptoms, and the intensified symptoms further discourage social interaction.

At the workplace, these dynamics manifest somewhat differently but are equally disruptive. The hallmark symptoms of SAD, such as difficulty concentrating, lethargy, and a general disinterest in work, can severely impact productivity and engagement. For many, this leads to a tangible decline in performance, which is particularly distressing in professions where peak productivity aligns with the winter months. The guilt of perceived underperformance adds an additional emotional burden, potentially exacerbating the symptoms of SAD. Moreover, the interpersonal aspects of work, such as teamwork and client interactions, can become fraught with challenges. The reduced patience and increased sensitivity to feedback that often come with SAD can impair professional relationships, complicating collaborative projects and day-to-day communications.

On an emotional level, the impact of SAD extends beyond the individual to touch the lives of their loved ones. Families and friends may struggle to understand the changes in behavior and mood, which can appear abrupt or unprovoked. The person who once lit up the room might now struggle to engage in light conversation, a shift that can be perplexing and distressing to those without an understanding of SAD. The guilt and frustration felt by those suffering from SAD, aware of their altered interactions yet feeling powerless to change them, further compound their emotional turmoil. It is not uncommon for relationships to be tested during these months, as both parties grapple with the disorder's ramifications.

Amid these challenges, finding effective coping strategies becomes paramount not just for those with SAD but also for their support networks. At the individual level, maintaining a structured daily routine can provide a sense of normalcy and control. This might include regular exercise, which has been shown to boost serotonin levels, and making a concerted effort to expose oneself to natural light, whether by spending time outdoors or strategically positioning oneself near windows during the day. Additionally, light therapy, a cornerstone treatment for SAD, involves regular, scheduled exposure to a light source that emits bright light mimicking natural sunlight, which can help regulate mood and improve energy levels.

For families and friends, understanding and patience are key. Recognizing the symptoms of SAD and the limitations they impose can foster empathy and reduce frustrations. Open communication about the disorder can help demystify the changes in behavior, making them less personal and a more recognized symptom of a medical condition. Planning social activities that are low-key and require minimal effort from the person with SAD can also be helpful. These might include watching a movie at home instead of going out to a theater or having a quiet night in with close friends rather than a large party. Moreover, encouraging and supporting the individual in their treatment—whether by reminding them to use their supplemental light therapy or accompanying them on walks—can be an integral part of the coping strategy, reinforcing the notion that they are not facing SAD alone.

In workplaces, accommodations can play a significant role in helping individuals manage SAD. Flexibility in work hours, especially during the darker months, or the option to work from home can significantly alleviate symptoms. Employers can also promote a supportive culture by fostering an environment where mental health is openly discussed and prioritized, which not only helps those with SAD but enhances the overall workplace environment. Providing information about SAD and training on mental health awareness can equip colleagues and supervisors with the tools to offer appropriate support, creating a more inclusive and understanding workspace.

As we navigate the complexities of SAD, recognizing its profound impact on social and professional spheres is significant. By adopting targeted coping strategies and fostering supportive environments, both at home and at work, we can mitigate the effects of SAD, enabling those affected to maintain their relationships and professional responsibilities. This holistic approach not only aids in managing the disorder but also in preserving the quality of life during the challenging winter months.

1.5 PERSONAL STORIES: LIVING WITH SAD FROM DIVERSE PERSPECTIVES

The human experience of Seasonal Affective Disorder manifests uniquely across different individuals, each narrative shedding light on the profound impact of this condition. Through a collection of personal stories, the stark reality of living with SAD becomes evident, as well as the resilience and adaptability it engenders. These narratives illustrate the challenges faced and highlight the diverse strategies employed to manage and overcome the disorder.

One compelling account comes from a middle-aged teacher from Minnesota, who noticed that each winter brought an inexplicable cloud over her life. The joy she felt in her work and her hobbies began to wane as daylight dwindled. Initially dismissing this as typical winter tiredness, it wasn't until she found herself struggling to leave her bed for days that she sought help and was diagnosed with SAD. Her story emphasizes the creeping nature of SAD and the importance of recognizing its symptoms early. Through a combination of light therapy and cognitive behavioral therapy, she learned to manage her symptoms. Her proactive approach allowed her to reclaim her winters, turning them from a time of dread to one of peaceful coexistence with her condition. Her experience underscores how personalized treatment plans can significantly restore one's quality of life.

On the familial front, the husband of a woman suffering from SAD shares his perspective, detailing the ripple effects of the disorder on their family dynamics. He shares the confusion and helplessness he initially felt watching his wife withdraw into herself each winter. His narrative is a poignant reminder of the emotional toll SAD can take on loved ones. However, through mutual learning and adaptation, including joining his wife for morning walks and helping her maintain a routine, they found a new rhythm for their relationship. His story highlights the important role of support and understanding from family, providing a scaffolding upon which individuals with SAD can lean when they feel most vulnerable.

In terms of overcoming challenges, a young artist from Washington recounts her journey with SAD, emphasizing the power of creative expression in her coping strategy. She describes how painting began as a form of escapism from the weight of her depression but gradually evolved into a therapeutic ritual that helped her process her emotions. Her studio, equipped with a light therapy lamp, became her sanctuary where she could simulate the much-needed daylight and immerse herself in her art. This creative outlet provided not just relief, but a sense of purpose during the months that had once been marked by despair. Her story is a testament to the therapeutic power of creativity and its ability to transform the burdensome into something beautiful and uplifting.

Community support also plays an important role in mitigating the isolation that can accompany SAD. An example of this is found in a community group in Alaska, where long winters profoundly affect a large portion of the population. The group, which started as a small support circle, quickly grew into a community-wide initiative, offering various activities and workshops designed to keep people engaged and socially connected throughout the harsh winters. From light therapy sessions to yoga classes designed to boost mood and energy, the group's activities are geared towards combating the common symptoms of SAD. The success of this community effort highlights the importance of collective action in creating environments that foster emotional well-being and resilience against seasonal depression.

These stories, each from a different vantage point, paint landscapes of life with SAD. They reveal the challenges and the triumphs, the personal struggles, and the communal victories. More importantly, they show that while SAD is a part of their lives, it does not define them. Through adaptive strategies, supportive relationships, and community engagement, individuals living with SAD continue to lead rich, fulfilling lives.

1.6 GENDER DIFFERENCES IN SAD: UNDERSTANDING THE DISPARITY

The question of why some individuals are more susceptible to Seasonal Affective Disorder (SAD) than others can often lead to a discussion about gender. Statistically, it is observed that women are more likely to be diagnosed with SAD than men, with some studies suggesting that as many as four women are affected for every one man. This significant disparity raises important questions about the underlying factors contributing to such differences, and how these insights shape our approach to treatment and support.

A primary area of interest in understanding why SAD affects more women than men lies in the realm of hormonal influences. The hormonal systems in women and men operate differently, and it is well-documented that hormones have a powerful influence on mood. For women, fluctuations in estrogen and progesterone throughout the menstrual cycle can significantly impact mood and have been linked to symptoms of depression in conditions such as premenstrual syndrome (PMS) and perimenopause. In the context of SAD, these hormonal fluctuations may interact with the physiological changes caused by reduced sunlight in the winter months, exacerbating mood disturbances and depressive symptoms. Estrogen, in particular, plays a role in regulating the neurotransmitters associated with mood, including serotonin. As daylight decreases during the fall and winter, the natural decline in serotonin may be more pronounced in women due to the concurrent fluctuations in estrogen levels, potentially increasing their vulnerability to SAD.

Moreover, the role of melatonin—a hormone that regulates sleep-wake cycles and is affected by changes in light exposure—also differs in its activity between genders. Research suggests that the production of melatonin is higher in women than in men, which could contribute to the increased sleepiness and lethargy associated with SAD. This difference in melatonin dynamics might explain why women are more likely to report the fatigue and energy loss that characterizes SAD, further complicating their day-to-day functioning during the winter months.

Beyond biological factors, social and cultural influences also play crucial roles in how SAD is experienced and managed across genders. Cultural norms and expectations can shape the way individuals express and respond to emotional distress. Women, often socialized to be more open about their feelings, might be more likely to seek help for mood disorders, leading to higher diagnosis rates. In contrast, men might underreport their symptoms due to prevailing norms that equate emotional expression with weakness. These cultural dynamics can affect not only the likelihood of being diagnosed with SAD but also the willingness to adhere to treatment. Understanding these social patterns is essential for developing supportive environments that encourage all individuals, regardless of gender, to seek help.

The recognition of these gender-specific factors necessitates a tailored approach to the treatment and support of individuals with SAD. It is imperative that healthcare providers consider these differences when developing management plans. For instance, treatment modalities might need to address the hormonal component more explicitly in women by considering the timing of light therapy in relation to menstrual cycles or exploring pharmacological options that take into account hormonal fluctuations. Similarly, psychoeducation and support structures for men with SAD might need to focus more on overcoming cultural stigmas associated with mental health and promoting healthier, more adaptive ways of expressing and managing emotions.

In addressing SAD, it is prudent to adopt a nuanced approach that not only recognizes the biological underpinnings of the disorder but also embraces the complex social and cultural landscapes in which individuals live. By integrating an understanding of gender disparities into our strategies for prevention, treatment, and support, we can enhance the effectiveness of our interventions and support all individuals in managing SAD more successfully. This tailored approach ensures that each person receives the understanding and care they need, reflecting a broader commitment to nuanced and empathetic healthcare.

2

TREATMENT AND MANAGEMENT STRATEGIES

A s the chill of winter sets in and the days grow shorter, many find themselves wrestling not just with the cold, but with the creeping shadows of Seasonal Affective Disorder (SAD). While the frosty weather calls for physical warmth, treating SAD demands a different kind of illumination—one that involves shedding light, quite literally, on effective management strategies. In this chapter, we delve into an array of treatments, beginning with one of the most validated and accessible interventions: light therapy.

2.1 LIGHT THERAPY DEMYSTIFIED: HOW IT WORKS AND FINDING YOUR SUPPLEMENTAL LIGHT SOURCE

Principles of Light Therapy

Imagine, if you will, the gloom of winter subtly encroaching upon your mood, your energy dwindling as the sunlight fades. Here is where light therapy, a cornerstone in the treatment of Seasonal

Affective Disorder, steps in as a beacon of relief. This therapy utilizes a specially designed light source, emitting a bright light that mimics the natural sunlight absent during the long winter months. The core idea is straightforward yet profound—by exposing yourself to this artificial sunlight, you can trick your brain into believing it's still basking in the vibrant days of summer.

The science behind light therapy hinges on its ability to simulate the effects of natural light on the brain, particularly targeting the regulation of two crucial hormones: melatonin and serotonin. As you might recall, the balance between these hormones is pivotal; where melatonin controls sleep cycles, serotonin uplifts mood. During the darker months, an increase in melatonin production can lead to lethargy and feelings of depression, a hallmark of SAD. Light therapy works by suppressing the daytime secretion of melatonin, thereby alleviating these symptoms. Furthermore, it helps maintain a healthy level of serotonin, bolstering your mood and fending off the depressive states induced by SAD.

Choosing Supplemental Light Source

Selecting the right light fixture, as one might surmise, is vital to the success of light therapy. There are several factors you should consider to ensure you reap the maximum benefits. First, is the intensity of the light, which is measured in lux. One lux (Latin for "light") is the amount of illumination provided when one lumen is evenly distributed over an area of one square meter. The lux of the light fixture should ideally be 10,000 lux, to effectively mimic the brightness of the sun. However, with greater intensity comes a shorter required exposure time, making it a convenient option for your morning routine. Some people get confused as some thera-peutic light fixtures are equipped to deliver, blue, red, white, and/or broad spectrum light. These fixtures may contain fluorescent or LED bulbs and filters to block UV rays. The red light spectrum is more for skin treatment, and reducing sleep inertia vs the white broad spectrum light which is commonly used for treatment of SAD.

Safety and the quality of light are paramount. A good light fixture will filter out UV rays, protecting your eyes and skin from potential harm. All that I researched on Amazon did have built in UV filters. Additionally, the type of light—broad-spectrum light is preferable—can affect the efficacy of the treatment, with some studies suggesting that certain spectrums might be more effective than others in treating SAD, depending on the individual. Cost is also a consideration. Some more expensive models may offer warranties, and additional features like adjustable angles, temperature, brightness, timers, remote control and memory. There are intermediate models and basic models that can be just as effective if they meet the necessary light intensity and safety standards.

Effective Use

Integrating light therapy into your daily routine can be seamless with a few strategic practices. For optimal results, light therapy should be used daily, especially during the months when you're most susceptible to SAD symptoms. Timing is significant— morning sessions are typically recommended because they help reset your circadian rhythm, mimicking the natural wake-up signals of sunrise. Positioning is also important. If you are using, a light box, it should be placed about 16 to 24 inches from your face, directly in your line of sight, ensuring you are not looking directly into the light, but receiving the light through your eyes, which is necessary for it to be effective. The length of time for the light exposure depends on the individual, and the intensity of the light. Many start with 20 to 30 minutes of light exposure in the morning and adjust from there. In chapter 7 I elaborate more on light therapy, as there are several styles and forms of supplemental therapeutic light such as head sets, visors, eye wear, floor lamps, desk lamps, table-top, box type and entire smart fixtures built into newer homes.

Evidence and Efficacy

Skeptical about flipping a switch to lift the gloom of winter depression? You're not alone. However, numerous studies bolster the efficacy of light therapy in treating SAD. Research indicates that light therapy can significantly reduce the symptoms of SAD, with many individuals reporting substantial improvement within just a few weeks of starting treatment. The effectiveness of light therapy can be comparable to that of antidepressant medication for several cases of SAD, but with fewer side effects. This makes it not only a powerful tool in your SAD management arsenal but also a gentle one.

In considering light therapy, you're opting for a treatment that has a robust backing in the scientific community and offers a non-invasive, drug-free method to improve your well-being during the winter months. As we continue exploring other treatments and management strategies for SAD, keep in mind the simplicity and effectiveness of light therapy as a foundation upon which many find significant relief from the clutches of seasonal depression.

2.2 PHARMACEUTICAL OPTIONS: A GUIDE TO ANTIDEPRESSANTS AND SAD

When exploring treatments for Seasonal Affective Disorder (SAD), the conversation often pivots toward the realm of pharmaceuticals, particularly antidepressants. These medications can play a beneficial role in ameliorating the depressive symptoms associated with SAD, due in large part to their ability to modulate neuro-transmitters that influence mood and emotional well-being. Among the most common and effective in treating SAD are the selective serotonin reuptake inhibitors (SSRIs). SSRIs work by blocking the reabsorption (reuptake) of serotonin in the brain, making more serotonin available to improve transmission of messages between neurons. This is particularly relevant in SAD, where diminished light leads to lower serotonin levels, contributing to mood deterioration.

The effectiveness of SSRIs in treating SAD is well-documented, with many patients reporting significant improvements in mood, energy levels, and overall outlook on life. Some examples of generic and brand name SSRI medications are: citalopram (Celexa), escitalopram (Lexapro), fluoxetine (Prozac, Sarafem), fluvoxamine (Luvox), paroxetine (Brisdelle, Paxil, Pexeva), sertraline (Zoloft), and vilazodone (Viibryd). However, the decision to use SSRIs—or any antidepressant—should not be taken lightly. These are potent medications that alter brain chemistry and can have a range of side effects, from mild (such as nausea, dizziness, drowsiness, diarrhea, constipation, and dry mouth) to more severe (such as fatigue, headaches, high blood pressure, tremors, seizures, agitation, and sexual dysfunction). The key to successfully incorporating SSRIs into the treatment of SAD lies in a personalized approach, guided by a knowledgeable healthcare provider who can navigate the complex landscape of antidepressant therapy with you.

Navigating the choices of medication requires a collaborative effort between you and your healthcare provider. The process typically begins with a comprehensive evaluation, including a detailed discussion of your symptoms, medical history, and any previous experiences with antidepressants. This information is vital, as it helps your doctor determine which medication is most likely to be effective and well-tolerated. Factors such as potential interactions with other medications you might be taking and any pre-existing health conditions like liver or kidney disease and allergies, will also influence this choice.

Once a medication has been selected, the next step is managing expectations and side effects. Starting an antidepressant can be an exercise in patience; it may take several weeks, sometimes longer, for the full effects to be experienced. During this period, monitoring and communication are key. Keeping a daily journal about how you are feeling as well as any pertinent changes in mood, weight, sleep patterns, or other symptoms and side effects, will be helpful. Regular follow-ups with your healthcare provider are essential to assess the effectiveness of the medication and make any necessary adjustments. Managing side effects, a common reason patients discontinue antidepressants prematurely, involves a strategic approach—sometimes an adjustment in dosage or a switch to a different medication can alleviate undesirable effects without sacrificing efficacy.

Medication should not be viewed as a standalone solution but rather as part of a comprehensive treatment plan that includes psychotherapy, lifestyle changes, light therapy, and possibly other treatment modalities like aroma therapy or acupuncture. The synergy between these different modalities can enhance overall effectiveness and provide more robust relief from SAD symptoms. For instance, while SSRIs can help correct the chemical imbalances in the brain, cognitive-behavioral therapy (CBT) can equip you with strategies to manage negative thought patterns associated with depression. Similarly, regular exercise, balanced wholesome nutrition, and a structured daily routine can further enhance your mood and general well-being, creating a multi-faceted approach that addresses SAD from several angles.

The journey through pharmaceutical options for SAD, particularly the use of SSRIs, is a nuanced path that requires careful consideration and management. By understanding the role these medications can play, actively participating in the choice and management of treatment, and integrating them into a broader strategy that includes other therapeutic approaches, you can significantly improve your quality of life during the challenging winter months. This integrated approach ensures that you are treating the symptoms and building a resilient foundation for long-term management and well-being.

2.3 PSYCHOTHERAPY FOR SAD: COGNITIVE BEHAVIORAL STRATEGIES

Cognitive Behavioral Therapy (CBT) stands as a beacon of hope for many grappling with Seasonal Affective Disorder (SAD), offering a structured, psychological approach to managing the condition. Unlike treatments that focus solely on the biological aspects of SAD, CBT addresses the psychological underpinnings by identifying and altering negative thought patterns and behaviors that can exacerbate or trigger depressive episodes during the darker months. This form of therapy is predicated assuming that our thoughts, feelings, and behaviors are interconnected, and that altering one can significantly impact the others, leading to improved mood and functionality.

At the core of CBT for SAD is the identification of negative thought patterns—often automatic, distorted thoughts about oneself and the environment that contribute to feelings of depression. For example, a common cognitive distortion among those with SAD might be overgeneralization, where one might conclude, based on a few gloomy days, that the entire winter will be miserable and unendurable. CBT works by challenging these automatic thoughts and replacing them with more balanced and realistic ones. This process, known as cognitive restructuring, involves keeping a daily log of negative thoughts, the emotions they provoke, and the contexts in which they occur. Over time, with the guidance of a therapist, you learn to recognize and dispute these distorted thoughts, gradually reshaping your cognitive landscape to one that is less conducive to depression and self empowering.

Additionally, CBT for SAD includes behavioral activation, a technique aimed at helping you engage more fully with life, particularly during the winter months when the inclination might be to withdraw and isolate. This might involve scheduling regular activities that encourage exposure to natural light, such as morning walks or sitting near a window during daylight hours. The premise here is simple yet powerful: by maintaining engagement with enjoyable activities, you can counteract the lethargy and withdrawal that are characteristic of SAD, thereby improving your overall mood and energy levels.

The effectiveness of CBT in treating SAD is well-supported by research. Numerous studies have shown that individuals who undergo CBT for SAD experience significant reductions in their depressive symptoms, often with lasting effects that extend beyond the winter season. One notable aspect of CBT's efficacy is its potential to not only treat current symptoms but also to provide skills and strategies that help prevent future episodes. This preventative aspect is particularly important in the context of SAD, which tends to recur seasonally. By learning effective coping strategies, you can better manage your mood each year as the seasons change, potentially reducing the severity and duration of future depressive episodes.

Finding a Therapist

Choosing the right therapist is an important step in successfully utilizing CBT to manage SAD. It's necessary to find a mental health professional who is trained in CBT and understands the unique challenges of SAD. When searching for a therapist, consider starting with referrals from your primary care provider or through reputable mental health organizations. Online directories of licensed therapists can also be a valuable resource, allowing you to filter potential therapists by specialty, insurance acceptance, and location.

When meeting with a potential therapist, don't hesitate to ask about their experience and success in treating SAD with CBT. Inquire about their approach to therapy, what a typical session might look like, and how they measure progress. It's also important to assess how comfortable you feel with the therapist; a strong therapeutic alliance—marked by trust, respect, and mutual understanding—is essential for effective therapy.

Engaging in CBT requires commitment and active participation, both in and out of therapy sessions. Your therapist will likely assign 'homework'—exercises and activities to practice the skills learned in therapy. These might include daily mood logs, structured schedules for activity and light exposure, and exercises in cognitive restructuring. Regularly practicing these techniques increases their efficacy and helps integrate them into your daily life, enhancing your ability to manage SAD effectively.

In summary, CBT offers a robust framework for understanding and tackling the cognitive and behavioral aspects of SAD. By focusing on modifying detrimental thought patterns and encouraging active engagement with life, CBT equips you with the tools to navigate the winter months more comfortably and to potentially lessen the impact of SAD in the future. As you continue exploring this therapeutic approach, remember that the journey to better mental health is a proactive one, requiring both insight and action. With the right strategies and support, it is entirely possible to reclaim your well-being and look forward to the change of seasons with renewed optimism and resilience.

2.4 LIFESTYLE ADJUSTMENTS: DIET, EXERCISE, AND SLEEP HYGIENE

In managing Seasonal Affective Disorder (SAD), incorporating specific lifestyle adjustments plays a significant role. These changes, encompassing diet, exercise, and sleep hygiene, are not just supplementary but often foundational to alleviating the symptoms of SAD. Each element interlinks with the other, creating a supportive structure that fosters better mental health during the challenging winter months.

Dietary Considerations

The profound impact of diet on mood and well-being is well-documented but often underemphasized in discussions about SAD. Certain nutrients have a significant influence on brain chemistry, particularly those that affect neurotransmitter function. Omega-3 fatty acids, for instance, are necessary for brain health, influencing the fluidity of cell membranes and playing a role in anti-inflammatory processes. Found in oily fish like salmon, mackerel, and sardines, as well as in flaxseeds and walnuts, omega-3s can enhance brain function and may help mitigate the depressive symptoms of SAD. Another vital nutrient is vitamin D, often dubbed the 'sunshine vitamin,' which can be scarce during the dark winter months. Low levels of vitamin D are associated with a higher risk of depression, making its supplementation potentially beneficial for those with SAD. While it is available in dietary sources like fortified milk and egg yolks, the primary source is sunlight, and thus, supplementation during winter could be particularly advantageous.

Integrating these nutrients into your daily diet can be both enjoyable and beneficial. Consider, for instance, starting your day with a smoothie that incorporates flaxseed oil or walnuts, or preparing a weekly salmon dish that satisfies your palate and fortifies your body against the mood fluctuations associated with SAD. It's about making mindful choices that boost your intake of mood-enhancing nutrients without feeling restrictive. Additionally, maintaining a balanced diet rich in fruits, vegetables, lean proteins, healthy fats, and whole grains can help stabilize blood sugar levels, which is paramount in managing mood swings and energy.

Exercise as Treatment

Regular physical activity is a powerful antidote to depression and a core component of managing SAD. Exercise promotes the release of endorphins, often known as 'feel-good' hormones, and helps regulate the body's sleep-wake cycle, which can be particularly beneficial for those struggling with SAD. The challenge during the colder months is maintaining an exercise routine when the weather and diminished daylight can be demotivating.

The key is to find activities that you enjoy and can feasibly be integrated into your routine. Indoor exercises, such as yoga, pilates, strength training, or home aerobic workouts, can be effective alternatives when it's too cold or dark to exercise outside. Additionally, if you can manage to get outdoors during daylight hours, even brief activities like walking or cycling can significantly boost your exposure to natural light, enhancing the benefits of exercise by synchronizing your circadian rhythms and improving mood.

Setting realistic goals cannot be understated. For instance, aiming for at least 30 minutes of moderate-intensity exercise most days of the week is a commendable goal. This could include activities like brisk walking, dancing, or any continuous activity that elevates your heart rate and allows you to still hold a conversation. It's also helpful to schedule exercise sessions in your calendar as appointments, a strategy that can increase your commitment to physical activity.

Sleep Hygiene

The interconnections between sleep, circadian rhythms, and SAD are particularly pronounced. The disruption of circadian rhythms, a core feature of SAD, often leads to significant sleep disturbances —either insomnia or hypersomnia (oversleeping). Improving sleep hygiene can help realign your biological clock and enhance both the quantity and quality of your sleep, which can mitigate some of the mood disruptions associated with SAD.

Establishing a regular sleep schedule is fundamental. Going to bed and waking up at the same time every day helps regulate your body's internal clock and can improve your sleep quality. Creating a bedtime routine that promotes relaxation can also be beneficial. This might include activities such as reading, taking a warm bath, or practicing relaxation exercises like deep breathing or meditation. It's also important to make your sleeping environment conducive to restful sleep. This includes maintaining a cool, comfortable temperature in the bedroom, using blackout curtains to block out light, and removing and turning off electronic devices that emit blue light. If, it is a necessity to use electronic devices that emit blue light after sunset, using eye wear that blocks the blue light which disrupts sleep patterns, can be beneficial.

Integrating Changes

Embracing these lifestyle adjustments requires a holistic approach. It's not about overhauling your life overnight but making incremental changes that collectively enhance your ability to manage SAD. Start small—perhaps by incorporating more omega-3 fatty acids into your diet or by introducing a 10-minute yoga routine into your morning. Gradually, as these become integrated into your lifestyle, the cumulative effect of these changes can significantly alleviate the symptoms of SAD. Remember, consistency is key. Regularly practicing good sleep hygiene, maintaining an active lifestyle, eating nutrient-rich foods, avoiding alcohol and caffeine, supplemental light therapy, psychotherapy, and staying properly hydrated, can transform your approach to managing SAD, turning the winter months from a time of dread into a period of tranquility and stability.

2.5 NATURAL SUPPLEMENTS AND VITAMINS FOR SAD SUPPORT

As you navigate the various treatment options for Seasonal Affective Disorder (SAD), it's essential to consider the role of natural supplements and vitamins. These can serve as valuable adjuncts to more conventional treatments, potentially enhancing your overall management strategy for SAD. Among the most discussed in this context are vitamin D, B vitamins, and omega-3 fatty acids. Each of these has been researched for their effects on mood and mental health, offering a complementary approach to alleviating the symptoms associated with SAD.

Vitamin D, often referred to as the sunshine vitamin, is pivotal as its production in the body is triggered by skin exposure to sunlight. During the winter months, when days are shorter and sunlight is sparse, vitamin D deficiency can become more prevalent, particularly in northern latitudes. This deficiency is linked to a variety of health issues, including a predisposition to depression and SAD. Supplementing with vitamin D can therefore be particularly beneficial in these months, potentially compensating for the lack of natural sunlight exposure. B vitamins, including folic acid, B6, and B12, also play beneficial roles in mental health. They are essential for the synthesis and proper functioning of neurotransmitters like serotonin and dopamine, which regulate mood. Deficiencies in these vitamins have been associated with increased feelings of depression and fatigue, which are symptomatic of SAD.

Omega-3 fatty acids, primarily found in fish oil, have been widely studied for their anti-inflammatory properties and their role in brain health. These fatty acids are integral to the structure and function of neuronal membranes. EPA and DHA, two types of omega-3s, are especially significant for cognitive function and emotional regulation. Research has suggested that omega-3 supplementation can help alleviate symptoms of depression and might be beneficial for those with SAD, particularly in regulating mood swings and improving emotional well-being.

The scientific backing for these supplements is robust yet nuanced. Numerous studies have explored the relationship between vitamin D levels and mood disorders, finding a correlation between low levels of vitamin D and increased incidence of depression and SAD. Similarly, clinical trials involving omega-3 supplements have shown promising results in the management of depression, including SAD. B vitamins have been the subject of various research studies that suggest their role in enhancing mood and mitigating symptoms of depression, though the results are often more mixed and suggest they may be most effective when used as part of a broader dietary and treatment strategy.

Despite the potential benefits, it's best to approach supplementation with caution. The integration of any supplement into your treatment plan should first be discussed with a healthcare provider. This is particularly important due to the potential for interactions with other medications and the risk of side effects. For example, excessive intake of vitamin D can lead to toxicity, with symptoms such as nausea, vomiting, and serious complications like kidney damage. Similarly, omega-3 supplements can interact with medications that affect blood clotting.

If you and your healthcare provider decide that adding supplements could be beneficial, integrating them into your daily routine requires thoughtful consideration. It's not merely about popping pills but ensuring these supplements fit synergistically into your broader health regimen. For instance, taking vitamin D with a meal that includes fat can improve its absorption, while B vitamins are generally more effective when taken as part of a comprehensive multivitamin/mineral supplement that provides a balanced range of nutrients necessary for their optimal function. Adding one new nutritional supplement at a time allows for isolating the benefits vs possible untoward side effects that you may experience.

Incorporating these supplements should be viewed as one component of a multifaceted approach to managing SAD. They are not a cure in themselves but can significantly bolster the effectiveness of other treatments such as light therapy, medication, and psychotherapy. By thoughtfully integrating natural supplements and vitamins into your lifestyle, guided by scientific evidence and professional advice, you enhance your ability to manage the symptoms of SAD, paving the way for a more balanced mood and improved overall well-being during the challenging winter months.

2.6 INNOVATIVE TREATMENTS: FROM AROMATHERAPY TO TMS

In the evolving landscape of treatments for Seasonal Affective Disorder (SAD), a spectrum of innovative therapies has emerged, broadening the horizon beyond traditional methods. Among these, aromatherapy, acupuncture, Transcranial Magnetic Stimulation (TMS), massage, mediation, and sound bowls or resonate frequencies represent a frontier of alternative approaches that cater to diverse patient needs and preferences. Each of these therapies offers unique mechanisms of action and potential benefits that could transform the management of SAD for many sufferers.

Aromatherapy, a practice that involves the use of essential oils derived from plants, proposes a gentle yet effective means of elevating mood and reducing stress and anxiety—common companions of SAD. The inhalation of these oils stimulates the olfactory system, the part of the brain connected to smell, which sends signals directly to the limbic system, the area of the brain responsible for emotions and memories. For instance, the aroma of lavender is widely recognized for its calming effects, while citrus scents like orange and bergamot can uplift the spirit and invigorate the senses. Although research into aromatherapy's efficacy for SAD specifically is still developing, preliminary studies suggest positive outcomes in reducing depressive symptoms, making it a compelling complementary treatment option.

Acupuncture, a traditional Chinese medicine technique that involves the insertion of thin needles into specific points on the body, is another modality gaining attention for its potential to alleviate symptoms of SAD. This practice is based on the belief that health is governed by the flow of Qi (vital energy) through the body, and that disruptions in this flow lead to illness, including mood disorders. By targeting specific acupuncture points associated with emotional health, practitioners aim to rebalance the body's energy, thereby improving mood and energy levels. Current research, while still in early stages, indicates that acupuncture can have a significant antidepressant effect, likely related to its ability to modulate neurotransmitters like serotonin and dopamine.

Transcranial Magnetic Stimulation (TMS) represents a more technologically advanced treatment option. This non-invasive procedure uses magnetic fields to stimulate nerve cells in the brain, with a focus on regions affected by depression. During a TMS session, an electromagnetic coil is placed against the scalp near the forehead, and short electromagnetic pulses are administered through the coil. The magnetic pulses induce small electric currents, which stimulate nerve cells in the region of the brain involved in mood regulation and depression. Notably, TMS has been shown to offer relief for patients who do not respond to traditional treatments, and its use in SAD is promising, given its direct action on the brain's mood circuits.

Sound bowls or other resonate frequencies have also been studied and found to have positive calming and healing benefits, such as the 528hz frequency for balancing and healing. One can find apps and social media platforms, such a YouTube, that offer a variety of formats in listening to specific frequencies of sound waves. There are also combination therapies such as massage therapy with healing sound frequencies and aroma therapy all in the same setting.

The anecdotal evidence from individuals who have explored these therapies often highlights profound benefits. For example, a person with SAD who found little relief from standard light therapy and medication might incorporate acupuncture as an alternative, discovering that the sessions help significantly in managing their symptoms, restoring a sense of normalcy and balance during the winter months. Similarly, someone else might integrate aromatherapy into their daily routine, using lavender oil in a diffuser each night to promote relaxation and better sleep, contributing to overall well-being during the SAD-prone seasons. With so many options for potential beneficial therapy, an individualized plan of care can be developed for your optimal health and well-being.

For those considering these innovative treatments, it is important to navigate this exploration with careful consideration of several factors. Cost can be a significant barrier, as treatments like TMS are often expensive and not always covered by insurance. Accessibility is another concern, as not all treatments are widely available in every area. Moreover, the necessity of working closely with healthcare professionals cannot be overstressed; it is essential to consult with your doctor or mental health professional to understand how these treatments might fit into your overall management plan for SAD. They can help assess the suitability of each option based on your specific symptoms, medical history, and treatment goals.

As we continue to expand our understanding and application of these innovative treatments, their potential to change lives remains clear. For many, these therapies could represent the turning point in their struggle with SAD, offering new hope and possibilities for relief. With ongoing research and increasing accessibility, the future for individuals battling SAD looks increasingly bright, underscored by a growing arsenal of therapeutic options tailored to meet their unique needs and preferences.

In summarizing, this chapter has unveiled a tapestry of traditional and cutting-edge treatments, each offering unique benefits and considerations. From the well-established impacts of light therapy and SSRIs to the emerging potential of TMS, acupuncture, resonate frequencies, massage, meditation, exercise, nutritional supplements, and aromatherapy, the landscape of SAD treatment is rich with options, allowing for personalized and effective management strategies. As we transition to the next chapter, we will explore the role of support systems and community resources in enhancing treatment outcomes and providing a network of care for those affected by SAD.

3

PERSONAL MANAGEMENT TECHNIQUES

A s the winter months draw near, it's not just the cold that sweeps through our homes but often a shadow that can chill the spirit: Seasonal Affective Disorder (SAD). While treatments like light therapy and medication are pivotal, as well as the other treatment modalities discussed, the environment where you spend your daily life—your sanctuary—plays an equally significant role in managing SAD. This chapter delves into how you can transform your living space into a bastion against the bleakness of winter, fostering a haven that not only brightens your space but also your mood.

3.1 CREATING A SAD-FRIENDLY HOME ENVIRONMENT

Maximizing Natural Light

The scarcity of sunlight during the winter months significantly contributes to the symptoms of SAD, making it essential to maximize whatever natural light is available. Start by examining the layout of your home—especially areas where you spend most of your time such as the living room or home office. Positioning furniture to take advantage of natural light can make a big difference. For instance, placing your desk or favorite reading chair near a window can provide direct exposure to natural light, boosting your mood and energy levels.

Window treatments can also play a beneficial role besides aesthetics and privacy. Opting for light-colored or translucent curtains can help maximize the penetration of natural light into your home. During daylight hours, make it a habit to pull back curtains and lift blinds completely, which invites more light into your space and connects you with the outdoors, reducing feelings of confinement and gloom. If privacy is a concern, consider using sheer fabrics that allow light to pass while still providing coverage.

Mood-Enhancing Decor

The colors and objects you surround yourself with can impact your mood. Color psychology suggests that certain colors evoke feelings of happiness and calm. For instance, shades of blue stimulate feelings of serenity and stability, greens are restful and soothing, and yellows can bring cheerful vibes into your home. Incorporate these colors through wall paint, pillow covers, rugs, or art pieces to create a visually therapeutic environment.

Plants are another wonderful addition to any home, especially for individuals dealing with SAD. Not only do they bring a touch of nature indoors, but they also have mood-boosting qualities. The act of nurturing a plant can itself be therapeutic and help foster a sense of accomplishment and connectivity. Choose low-maintenance indoor plants such as spider plants, peace lilies, succulents, or philodendrons, which thrive indoors with minimal sunlight.

Creating Relaxation Spaces

Dedicating a specific area of your home for relaxation and mindfulness can be a sanctuary from the stressors of daily life and the intrusive symptoms of SAD. This could be a corner of your bedroom or a part of your living room where you can meditate, practice yoga, or simply sit quietly and reflect. Equip this space with elements that promote relaxation—comfortable seating like a bean bag, yoga mat or a soft rug, calming scents from candles or essential oils, and perhaps soothing sounds of white noise, rain, the ocean, resonate frequencies, or even a small indoor fountain.

Lighting Solutions

Beyond the use of natural light, artificial lighting solutions can also play a significant role in combating the symptoms of SAD. Light therapy lamps are a well-known remedy, but their usage can extend beyond structured therapy sessions. Integrating these lamps into your home decor can provide continued exposure to mood-boosting light. For example, placing a light therapy lamp in your relaxation area or on your work desk can provide ongoing benefits throughout the day.

Additionally, consider the color temperature of the lighting in your home. Warm white bulbs tend to provide a cozy, comforting glow, making evening environments more relaxing. However, during the day, bulbs mimicking daylight with a cooler blue-white hue can be more energizing and better simulate the effects of natural daylight.

Transforming your living space into a supportive environment doesn't require a complete overhaul—simple adjustments can significantly enhance your comfort and well-being. By maximizing natural light, incorporating mood-enhancing elements, creating dedicated relaxation spaces, and utilizing strategic lighting solutions, you can create a home that shelters you physically and supports your mental health through the challenging winter months. This proactive approach to managing your environment empowers you to create a space that combats the symptoms of SAD and transforms your home into a source of comfort and joy, in any season.

3.2 ROUTINE BUILDING: STRUCTURING YOUR DAY FOR BETTER MOOD STABILITY

Establishing a consistent daily routine is akin to setting the tempo for a symphony—it brings harmony and rhythm to your life, especially when navigating the ebb and flow of Seasonal Affective Disorder (SAD). The predictability of a well-structured day can significantly mitigate the disarray brought on by SAD, anchoring your biological clock to a steady beat, which in turn regulates mood and energy levels. By crafting a routine that harmonizes key elements such as light exposure, exercise, nutrition, and relaxation, you create a daily cadence that supports your mental, emotional, and physical well-being.

Consider the profound impact that a morning routine can have when tailored to counteract SAD. Start with choosing a positive mindset/intention, then light exposure; if natural sunlight is scarce, a light therapy session first thing in the morning can fill that void. Integrating this into your morning ritual can help suppress the excess melatonin that makes you groggy and dispirited. Follow this with a wholesome breakfast, then a simple exercise routine, which could be a series of stretching exercises and/or a brisk indoor workout. This physical activity kickstarts your endorphin levels, boosting your mood and energy. Cap off your morning routine with a mindfulness practice, such as meditation, prayer, and/or journaling. This helps in grounding your thoughts and sets a positive tone for the day.

Transitioning into the afternoon, maintain your momentum by aligning meal times and work tasks with your energy levels. A well-timed, nutritious lunch serves as both a physical and mental break, replenishing your body and dividing your day into manageable segments. Post-lunch, when energy often dips, schedule less demanding tasks or those that offer variety and engagement to combat fatigue. The key is to adapt your tasks to your fluctuating energy levels, which are part of the SAD experience, thereby maintaining productivity without overwhelming yourself. Of course, adequate hydration should not be overlooked.

As evening approaches, prepare for a tranquil transition to rest. Dim the lights to cue your body for sleep, reflecting the natural progression from daylight to dusk. Engage in relaxing activities such as reading, listening to soft music, or a gentle yoga session. These activities not only ease the transition into sleep but also combat the intrusive thoughts and worries that often accompany SAD. This structured wind-down routine plays a helpful role in enhancing your sleep quality, paramount for mood regulation and overall health.

Tools and Resources

To effectively maintain such a routine, especially when SAD which can cloud motivation and energy, leveraging the right tools and resources is essential. Numerous apps and planning tools are available to help you structure and adhere to your daily routine. Apps like "Calm" or "Headspace" offer guided mindfulness and meditation sessions that can easily fit into any part of your day, supporting your mental health. For physical activity, apps like "MyFitnessPal" or "Yoga Studio" provide customizable exercise options that can be adapted to indoor environments, catering to the days when leaving home feels daunting.

Furthermore, routine-building tools like "Google Calendar" or "Todoist" allow you to visually map out your day, set reminders, and track your progress, reinforcing your daily and seasonal routines. These tools can be particularly helpful in maintaining consistency, a key challenge for those experiencing SAD. They offer the flexibility to adjust your schedule as needed, accommodating the good days and the tough ones, thus supporting a responsive approach to managing your symptoms.

By embracing these strategies and tools, you empower yourself to build and maintain a daily routine that navigates the challenges of SAD and enhances your overall quality of life. It's about creating a framework that supports your well-being, enabling you to handle the fluctuations of your symptoms with grace and efficiency. Through a well-considered routine, each day can be met with renewed strength and optimism, making SAD a manageable part of life rather than an overwhelming one. This proactive approach to structuring your day ensures that despite the shorter, darker days, your life retains its light and rhythm.

3.3 THE ROLE OF MINDFULNESS AND MEDITATION IN MANAGING SAD

Mindfulness Basics

In the quiet moments of the morning, as the world still lingers in the soft embrace of dawn, there exists a profound opportunity for transformation. This is the essence of mindfulness—a practice rooted in the here and now, focusing wholly on the present moment. For those facing Seasonal Affective Disorder (SAD), mindfulness offers more than just a respite; it provides a powerful tool to recalibrate the mind's response to the external gloom imposed by the season. At its core, mindfulness involves observing your current experiences without judgment—acknowledging thoughts, feelings, and sensations as they arise and letting them pass without attachment.

The relevance of mindfulness in managing mood disorders like SAD lies in its ability to alter the typical patterns of negative thinking that can exacerbate feelings of depression. By training yourself to remain present and engaged with the immediate environment, you gradually decrease the prevalence of ruminative thoughts that often dominate the landscape of SAD. This shift in focus can lead to significant changes in how you perceive and react to the daily challenges posed by the disorder. For instance, instead of being overwhelmed by a day of overcast sky and frigid air, mindfulness encourages an acceptance of these conditions without allowing them to dictate your emotional state. The practice fosters a resilience that is both subtle and powerful, allowing you to encounter each day with a renewed sense of clarity and balance.

Meditation Techniques

Meditation, often a cornerstone of mindfulness practice, offers specific techniques that can be particularly beneficial for individuals with SAD. One such technique is focused attention meditation, which involves concentrating on a single point of interest, such as your breath or a specific sound. This practice not only helps in cultivating concentration but also serves as a training ground for directing your attention away from the cyclic patterns of depressive thoughts.

Another accessible technique for beginners is the body scan meditation. This involves mentally scanning your body from head to toe, noting any sensations of tension or discomfort without attempting to change them. This practice not only increases bodily awareness but also highlights how often our physical states are reflections of our mental battles, providing insights that are particularly valuable for those managing SAD.

For those particularly affected by the lack of light and color during the winter months, visualization meditation can be a soothing alternative. In this practice, you are guided to visualize a serene environment or a sunny day. The mental imagery can evoke the sensory experiences associated with these visuals, such as warmth or light, providing a mental escape from the dreariness of winter.

Integrating Mindfulness

Incorporating mindfulness into daily life can start with simple practices like mindful eating or walking meditation. Mindful eating involves paying close attention to the process of eating—observing the colors, textures, and flavors of your food, incorporating gratitude, and noticing how they affect your senses. This practice enhances your dining experience and improves your connection with food as a source of nourishment rather than just consumption.

Walking meditation is another practical approach, especially beneficial for those with SAD who might find it challenging to sit still. It involves walking slowly and deliberately, with full awareness of each step and the sensations of your feet touching the ground, the air you breathe and your surroundings. This can be particularly therapeutic when done outdoors, allowing for the dual benefits of mindfulness and mild exposure to natural light, even on overcast days. I wrote a little booklet called "Walking Meditation Using Chakras, Guide to Revitalizing and Balancing your Energy" which is available on Amazon. It is a practice that I do myself, and I thought it might help others in developing their own mindfulness practice.

Evidence of Benefits

The efficacy of mindfulness and meditation in alleviating symptoms of SAD is supported by a growing body of scientific research. Studies have shown that a regular mindfulness practice can lead to reductions in anxiety and depression, with improvements in mood and well-being that are comparable to those achieved through traditional psychotherapy or medication. For SAD sufferers, these benefits are often manifested in enhanced mood stability, increased energy levels, and improved sleep patterns, all of which are foundational for managing the disorder effectively.

The compelling aspect of mindfulness and meditation lies in their ability to transform the winter months from a time of dread to a period of potential growth and self-discovery. These practices equip you with the tools to navigate the challenges of SAD not by changing the external environment but by reshaping your internal landscape. With each mindful breath and meditative moment, you forge a path toward a more balanced and fulfilling winter season, proving that even in the darkest months, there is potential for light.

3.4 KEEPING ACTIVE: INDOOR EXERCISE ROUTINES FOR DARKER MONTHS

The profound connection between physical activity and mood enhancement is particularly significant for individuals managing Seasonal Affective Disorder (SAD). Engaging in regular exercise triggers a cascade of biochemical reactions in the brain, including the release of endorphins—often termed 'feel-good' hormones.

These natural mood lifters play an important role in alleviating the symptoms of depression associated with SAD. Moreover, exercise stimulates the production of serotonin and dopamine, neurotransmitters that are integral in regulating mood, sleep, and cognition. Thus, establishing a routine that includes physical activity can be a game-changer in managing the emotional challenges brought on by the shorter, darker days of winter.

However, the cold weather and limited daylight can make outdoor activities less appealing and sometimes impractical. This is where indoor exercises come into play, offering a viable alternative that ensures you stay active and uplift your spirits, regardless of the weather outside. A variety of indoor exercise options are available that cater to different interests and fitness levels, making it easier to find something that resonates with your lifestyle and preferences. For instance, aerobic exercises such as dancing, stationary cycling, or using a treadmill can significantly boost your heart rate and enhance your endorphin levels. These activities improve your physical health and have a rapid impact on lifting your mood.

Strength training is another excellent option that can be easily adapted for indoor settings. Activities like body-weight-resistance exercises, yoga, and pilates not only strengthen your muscles but also improve your body awareness and control, which can be incredibly empowering for someone dealing with mood fluctuations. The focus required for these exercises also helps divert your mind from negative thoughts, a common struggle for those experiencing SAD.

For those who prefer more structured exercise, online fitness classes can be a great resource. Many platforms offer a range of activities, from guided yoga and pilates sessions to more intense cardio workouts. These classes provide the flexibility to choose your workout style and intensity, fitting seamlessly into your schedule. Moreover, many come with the added benefit of a virtual community, which can be particularly motivating during times when isolation feels overpowering.

Maintaining motivation for regular exercise can be a hurdle, especially when your energy levels and mood are affected by SAD. Setting realistic goals is a fundamental strategy to keep yourself engaged. It's important to acknowledge that your energy levels will vary, and setting flexible, achievable targets can help maintain a positive perspective towards exercise. For example, committing to a 10-minute yoga session daily is a small, manageable goal that can gradually be increased as your energy and mood improve.

Finding an exercise buddy or joining a virtual workout group can also provide a significant motivational boost. The camaraderie and sense of accountability that come from working out with others can make it easier to stick to your exercise routine. Additionally, sharing your experiences and challenges with others who might be facing similar struggles provides emotional support, making the journey less daunting.

Community resources play an exciting role in supporting your indoor exercise routine. Many community centers and health clubs offer indoor classes that cater to those affected by seasonal changes. These programs are often designed with the understanding of the needs of individuals experiencing SAD, providing not just exercise guidance but also a supportive community environment. Additionally, local sports leagues or fitness challenges can offer a more competitive yet fun element to your exercise routine, which can be incredibly stimulating and rewarding. One example of a sports league that is growing nationwide is Pickleball. Many communities have both indoor and out door courts for Pickleball.

By integrating these indoor exercises into your daily routine, you create a robust framework to help manage SAD. The blend of endorphin-boosting workouts and the supportive structure of online or community resources provides a balanced approach to maintaining your physical and mental health during the winter months. This proactive strategy helps in managing the current symptoms and empowers you to take control of your well-being, transforming the winter season from a time of dread to a period of active engagement and personal growth.

3.5 NUTRITION AND MOOD: FOODS THAT FIGHT THE WINTER BLUES

Diet-Mood Connection

When winter rolls in, bringing darker days and colder temperatures, it's not just your wardrobe that needs adjusting but potentially your diet too, especially if you're battling Seasonal Affective Disorder (SAD). The foods you consume play a dramatic role in how you feel, both physically and emotionally. This is because certain nutrients have direct pathways influencing brain chemistry, impacting neurotransmitters that govern mood, energy levels, and even cognitive functions. For instance, amino acids found in protein sources are precursors to neurotransmitters like serotonin, and dopamine which is often dubbed the 'feel-good' hormone. Low levels of serotonin are linked to depression, which is why diets lacking in essential nutrients can exacerbate the symptoms of SAD.

Furthermore, complex carbohydrates are huge in influencing mood. They aid in the production of serotonin and help stabilize blood sugar levels, preventing the spikes and dips that can affect your energy and mood. On the other hand, simple carbohydrates, such as those found in sugary snacks and drinks, can lead to quick energy crashes that deepen mood swings. This intricate dance between what you eat and how you feel forms the foundation of using nutritional intake as a tool to combat SAD, making thoughtful dietary choices a powerful ally in managing the condition.

Mood-Boosting Foods

Incorporating mood-boosting foods into your diet can be a delicious and natural way to help manage the symptoms of SAD. Foods rich in Omega-3 fatty acids, such as salmon, walnuts, and flaxseeds, are top of the list. Omega-3s are essential fats that your body can't make but are foundational for brain health, impacting mood and cognitive function. They are thought to enhance the structures of brain cells necessary for neurotransmission, which can improve the symptoms of depression and SAD.

Another group of mood-enhancing foods includes those rich in B vitamins. These vitamins, particularly B12, B6, and folate, play profound roles in the production and regulation of neurotransmitters like serotonin and dopamine. Foods high in these vitamins include lean meats, eggs, leafy greens, and legumes. Regular consumption of these can help ensure your neurotransmitter levels are balanced, aiding in mood stabilization throughout the darker months.

Moreover, incorporating plenty of fresh vegetables and some fruits in your diet can contribute to better mood regulation. These foods are high in fiber, which helps slow the absorption of glucose into your bloodstream and prevents mood swings. They are also packed with antioxidants, which combat oxidative stress in the brain, potentially lowering the risk of depression. Brightly colored vegetables and fruits, such as berries, oranges, and carrots, are not only visually uplifting but also provide the nutrients necessary to boost your mood and overall health.

Meal Planning Tips

To effectively incorporate these mood-boosting foods into your daily diet, strategic meal planning is helpful. Start by creating a balanced weekly menu that includes a variety of nutrient-rich foods. Ensure each meal has a good source of protein, a complex carbohydrate, and plenty of fruits and vegetables. This balance supports overall health and ensures a steady supply of the nutrients needed to combat the symptoms of SAD.

Prepping meals in advance can also help you stick to your dietary plan, especially on days when your mood and energy might be lagging. Consider preparing large batches of meals that can be easily reheated throughout the week, or chopping and storing vegetables and fruits for quick snacks. This saves time and makes it more likely that you'll reach for healthy options.

Finally, try to set regular meal times. Eating at consistent times each day can help regulate your body's clock, which is often disrupted in SAD. Regular meal times can also stabilize blood sugar levels throughout the day, preventing mood dips and spikes.

Avoiding Pitfalls

While adjusting your diet to combat SAD, it's important to be aware of common dietary pitfalls that can undermine your efforts. High on the list are caffeine and sugar, which can provide temporary boosts but often lead to crashes that exacerbate mood swings and fatigue. Try to limit your intake of caffeinated beverages and opt for herbal teas instead, which can be soothing without the stimulating effects. Similarly, steer clear of sugary snacks and desserts that can lead to rapid changes in blood sugar levels, impacting your mood and energy levels.

Instead, focus on whole foods that provide sustained energy. Snacks like nuts, yogurt, or some fruit can offer the necessary nutrients without the negative side effects of caffeine or empty calories of sugar. By making these mindful choices, you can help stabilize your mood and energy throughout the winter months, making SAD more manageable and your days brighter and more enjoyable.

3.6 SLEEP STRATEGIES: COMBATTING THE SLEEP-WAKE CYCLE DISRUPTION

The intricate dance between our internal clocks and the environment is delicately balanced, and yet, for those grappling with Seasonal Affective Disorder (SAD), this balance is often disrupted, leading to significant sleep challenges. These disruptions manifest as difficulties in falling asleep, staying asleep, or waking earlier than desired, all of which can exacerbate the symptoms of SAD. Understanding and addressing these sleep issues is important for alleviating immediate discomfort and for maintaining overall health and well-being during the winter months.

Effective sleep hygiene practices tailored specifically to those with SAD can be transformative. It begins with establishing a consistent sleep schedule. Going to bed and waking at the same time every day, even on weekends, helps to regulate your body's internal clock, or circadian rhythm, which can be particularly erratic during the darker months. Avoiding stimulants like caffeine and nicotine close to bedtime ensures that your body's natural sleep readiness isn't hijacked. Similarly, while alcohol might seem like a way to ease into sleep, it actually disrupts sleep cycles, leading to a less restful night. Perhaps less obvious is the impact of electronic devices before bedtime; the blue light emitted by screens can significantly inhibit the production of melatonin, the hormone that signals your body to prepare for sleep. Therefore, setting a digital curfew an hour before bedtime can help enhance your sleep quality.

Creating a bedtime ritual is another effective strategy. Engaging in relaxing activities such as reading a book, taking a warm bath, or listening to calming music can signal to your body that it's time to wind down. These activities assist in the transition into sleep and help in distancing from the day's stresses, which can be harder to shake off during the depressive phases of SAD. Furthermore, incorporating relaxation techniques such as deep breathing exercises, progressive muscle relaxation, or meditation can actively combat the tension and anxiety that often accompany SAD, smoothing the path to restful sleep. For example, after taking a soothing bath/shower, lie down with eyes closed, inhale deeply, holding breath for a few moments while focusing on gratitude, then exhale slowly. Repeating this several times until you feel ready to start your mediation.

Bedroom Environment

The environment in which you sleep can greatly influence the quality of your rest. Optimizing your bedroom to make it conducive to sleep is therefore essential. The role of light in SAD makes it particularly important to manage light exposure in the bedroom. Using blackout curtains to eliminate light can help maintain darkness throughout the night, especially in urban settings where artificial lighting is prevalent. On the other hand, if waking up is a struggle, timed light therapy lamps that simulate sunrise can gently coax your body awake, aligning with natural circadian rhythms.

Temperature also plays an important role in sleep quality. A cooler room, typically around 65 degrees Fahrenheit, is often recommended as it supports the body's natural drop in temperature that occurs during sleep. Ensuring your bedding and sleepwear are comfortable and appropriate for the season can also prevent disruptions due to being too hot or too cold during the night.

Minimizing noise disruptions is another key aspect. While you may not have control over all external noises, tools like ear plugs, apps that play white noise, relaxing sounds of nature like that of rain or the ocean, may also be helpful in masking disruptive sounds. Additionally, keeping your bedroom exclusively for sleep and intimacy, rather than a space for work or entertainment, can strengthen the mental association between your bedroom and sleep, making it easier to relax and fall asleep each night.

When to Seek Help

Recognizing when sleep disruptions require professional intervention is important. If you've implemented sleep hygiene practices and optimized your sleep environment but still struggle with sleep quality or duration, it may be time to consult a healthcare provider. Persistent difficulties in falling or staying asleep, frequent awakenings during the night, or feeling unrefreshed despite a full night's sleep are signs that professional help might be needed. These sleep issues can be symptomatic of an underlying sleep disorder such as sleep apnea, or an indication that your SAD treatment needs adjustment.

Healthcare professionals can offer a range of solutions, from adjusting your current SAD treatments to exploring options like cognitive behavioral therapy for insomnia (CBT-I), a highly effective treatment that can be particularly beneficial for those whose sleep issues are compounded by SAD. Seeking help addresses the underlying problem, immediate discomfort and mitigates the long-term risks associated with poor sleep, such as impaired cognitive function, mood disturbances, and decreased immunity.

By understanding and addressing the sleep challenges associated with SAD, you can significantly enhance your quality of life during the winter months. Effective sleep strategies can improve night-time restorative rest, help stabilize mood, increase energy levels during the day, and strengthen overall resilience to SAD. As we continue to explore the multifaceted approaches to managing SAD in the following chapters, remember that each step taken to improve sleep is a step toward reclaiming your well-being and vitality throughout the season.

4

FOR FAMILY AND FRIENDS

When the short days and long nights of winter set in, not only do those with Seasonal Affective Disorder (SAD) feel the weight of the season, but so too do their loved ones. Understanding and addressing SAD within family dynamics and friendships is not just about providing support; it's about transforming understanding and empathy into actionable care that respects both the individual's experience and the collective well-being of the group. This chapter is dedicated to those who stand by, ready to lend support, offering them tools and insights to navigate the complexities of SAD with love, grace and effectiveness.

4.1 HOW TO TALK ABOUT SAD: APPROACHING SENSITIVE CONVERSATIONS

Initiating a dialogue about SAD with someone you care about can feel like walking a tightrope. On one side, there's the risk of sounding too intrusive or presumptive, and on the other, there's the fear of seeming indifferent or dismissive. Maintaining balance lies in choosing the right moment, framing your concerns with empathy, and fostering an environment of openness and trust. Timing is paramount; it's often most effective to start these conversations when the person feels comfortable and is in a relatively good state, rather than during a moment of distress. This timing ensures that your loved one is more likely to be receptive and that the conversation will be productive.

Empathy is your most powerful tool in this dialogue. It involves more than understanding what your loved one is going through; it's about showing them that their feelings are valid and that their experiences are real and significant to you. Start the conversation gently, perhaps by sharing what you've observed in a non-judgmental way. For example, you might say, "I've noticed you seem really down during the winter months, and I read that this can be a sign of Seasonal Affective Disorder. Would you like to talk about what you're feeling?" This approach is not confrontational but shows that you care and are paying attention, which can make all the difference.

Active listening is foundational once the conversation begins. This means truly hearing what your loved one is saying and responding in a way that confirms their feelings are heard. Active listening involves making eye contact, nodding, and occasionally paraphrasing what the person has said to ensure understanding. It's about creating a safe space where the person feels they can share their thoughts and feelings without fear of judgment or immediate solutions being thrown at them.

Educating yourself and others about SAD is another vital component. Misconceptions about SAD abound, and these can lead to stigma or minimization of the disorder ("It's just the winter blues!"). Take the time to learn about SAD from reliable sources, and gently share this information with others who might influence your loved one's environment. Education can dismantle myths and foster a supportive network that understands and validates the experience of living with SAD.

Lastly, handling resistance is part of the process. Not everyone is ready to talk about their mental health, nor will they always accept the perspective that what they're experiencing could be a form of depression. If your loved one is resistant or in denial about their symptoms, be patient. Emphasize that your primary concern is their happiness and well-being and that professional help is not about labeling them but offering support and relief. Sometimes, simply knowing that support is available and that you'll be there when they're ready to talk can be enough for now.

Interactive Element: Reflection Section

To aid in applying these conversation strategies, consider reflecting on the following questions after your discussions about SAD:

- How did the person react when you brought up your observations?
- What listening techniques did you find most effective?
- How can you continue to foster open communication about their feelings and experiences?

Taking the time to reflect on these interactions and, possibly, keeping a written journal, can improve your approach and understanding, making each conversation more thoughtful and supportive. This reflective practice can enhance your ability to support your loved and deepen your relationship, making it a source of comfort and strength for both of you during the winter months and beyond.

4.2 BEING AN EFFECTIVE PART OF A SUPPORT SYSTEM

When you commit to supporting someone with Seasonal Affective Disorder (SAD), understanding the multifaceted role you play is of utmost importance. A support system isn't just about providing comfort; it encompasses a range of roles and responsibilities that require careful navigation to ensure they're effective without being overwhelming. Establishing and respecting boundaries is perhaps the first, and most important, step in this process. It's vital to discuss and agree on what kind of support will be helpful and when it might be needed. This conversation helps in setting limits and boundaries that protect both your well-being and that of your loved one, preventing dependency, which can sometimes lead to resentment or burnout. For instance, you might agree to check in daily during the winter months, but not necessarily have long conversations every day unless they're needed. This helps in maintaining a balance where support is readily available without encroaching on personal space.

Providing practical support can take many forms and needs to be tailored to what the person with SAD finds most helpful. It could be as simple as helping them maintain a routine that includes exposure to natural light or assisting in managing medication schedules. Daily check-ins can be part of this, where a simple message asking how they are or reminding them about their medication can make a significant difference. On days when leaving the house feels daunting for them, offering to accompany them on a walk or a trip to the store can provide the necessary motivation and also ensure they get some exposure to natural light, which is beneficial in managing SAD.

Emotional support is equally important. It involves being there to listen, without judgment or the rush to offer solutions. Validating their feelings by acknowledging that what they're experiencing is tough and that it's okay to feel overwhelmed sometimes helps in making them feel understood. Encouragement plays a crucial role here; reminding them of their strengths and past successes in managing difficult days can boost their morale. For instance, recalling a day when they managed to go out despite feeling low and how good they felt after they went out, can be a powerful reminder of their ability to overcome challenging moments.

Another key aspect of being an effective support system is educating other friends and family about SAD. This helps in extending the support network and ensures that others' interactions with the person do not inadvertently make their symptoms worse. Misconceptions about SAD can lead to comments that might be well-intentioned but are actually harmful, like minimizing their feelings or pushing them too hard to 'snap out of it'. Educating those around you can involve sharing articles, resources, or even organizing a casual meet-up where the person with SAD feels comfortable discussing their experience. This facilitates broadening understanding and fosters a community of support, making the person with SAD feel less isolated and more supported.

Navigating these roles requires a delicate balance of care, respect, and communication. It's about being present and proactive in your support, but also stepping back when needed to allow space for independence. Each act of support, whether practical or emotional, contributes to a stronger, more resilient network, capable of withstanding the challenges of SAD, and ensuring that both you and your loved one find this support system to be a source of genuine comfort and effective aid. As you continue to build this system, remember that every small effort counts, and collectively, these efforts weave a safety net that holds strong against the weight of Seasonal Affective Disorder.

4.3 RECOGNIZING AND RESPONDING TO SAD-RELATED CRISES

When caring for someone with Seasonal Affective Disorder (SAD), it's imperative to recognize that while many can manage their symptoms adequately with routine treatments and support, some may experience severe episodes that can escalate into crises. These critical moments, characterized by acute depression or even thoughts of self-harm, require immediate and careful intervention. Recognizing these signs early can be the key to preventing a full-blown crisis. It often begins with noticeable changes in behavior; your loved one may suddenly seem overwhelmingly despondent, withdraw from social interactions more severely than usual, or express feelings of hopelessness or worthlessness. They might neglect their personal care, or you might notice significant disturbances in their sleep patterns, appetite, or overall demeanor. More alarming signs include verbal hints or outright declarations of self-harm or a preoccupation with death or dying. These indicators demand prompt attention and action to safeguard their well-being.

When you discern any of these acute signs, the first and most immediate step is to ensure the safety of your loved one. If there is any indication of self-harm or suicidal thoughts, it's necessary to act swiftly—remove any means of self-harm from the vicinity and stay with them or have someone they trust do so. Contacting a mental health professional immediately or seeking emergency medical help can be crucial. In these moments, clear, calm, and direct communication is vital. Express your concerns and the seriousness of the situation without panic, reassuring them of your support and the availability of help. It's essential to convey not just your readiness to assist them in getting the help they need but also your belief in their ability to recover, which can provide a glimmer of hope in a moment of deep despair.

Beyond the immediacy of crisis management, developing long-term strategies to prevent future crises is a must. This involves regular discussions with healthcare providers to ensure that the treatment plan is effective and adhered to, adjusting medications or therapies as needed. Establishing a proactive plan for managing future depressive episodes can also be beneficial. This might include identifying early warning signs together, creating a list of actionable steps to take when symptoms begin to escalate, and maintaining a list of emergency contacts such as their therapist, close family members, or a dedicated crisis hotline. Additionally, ensure that your loved one is connected to a supportive community, whether it's a therapy group, online support networks, or close friends and family who understand their condition and can offer immediate support when needed.

Supporting someone through the recovery phase post-crisis is equally important. This period can be fraught with vulnerability and confusion, making your patient, consistent support the foundation. Recovery is rarely linear, and understanding this can help you provide the compassionate support needed. Encourage open discussions about their feelings and experiences, and be vigilant for any signs of relapse. Regularly visiting and possibly revising their coping strategies can empower them, providing a sense of control and involvement in their own path to recovery. It's also a time to reaffirm the importance of continued therapy, whether it involves regular counseling sessions and/or medication management, and to reinforce the lifestyle strategies that support their overall well-being. This might include ensuring regular physical activity, adequate sleep, and nutrition, all of which play a significant role in mental health.

Navigating a crisis related to SAD can be challenging and intense, not just for the individual experiencing it but also for those around them. By understanding the signs of a crisis, knowing how to respond effectively, and implementing strategies to manage and recover from these episodes, you can provide a lifeline during these critical times. Your role in such instances is not just about immediate intervention but also about fostering an environment of ongoing support and recovery, helping your loved one not only to survive the winter months but to potentially emerge stronger and more resilient. Through careful preparation and responsive care, you help create a safer, more supportive space for dealing with SAD, making a profound difference in the life of someone facing this formidable challenge.

4.4 SUPPORTING THROUGH TREATMENT: TIPS FOR FAMILY AND FRIENDS

Navigating the treatment landscape for Seasonal Affective Disorder (SAD) can be as daunting for family and friends as it is for the person experiencing it. By gaining a clear understanding of the various treatment options available, you stand in a better position to offer informed and empathetic support. As we've discussed throughout this book, treatments for SAD range from light therapy, often the first line of treatment, to medication such as antidepressants, psychotherapies including cognitive behavioral therapy tailored for SAD (CBT-SAD), and much more. Each treatment has its own mechanism of action, benefits, and considerations. For instance, light therapy involves exposure to a bright light that mimics natural sunlight, which can help regulate the body's sleep-wake cycle and mood. Understanding these details allows you to engage in meaningful discussions about the treatments' purposes and effects, fostering a supportive environment where the person with SAD feels empowered to adhere to their treatment regimen.

Accompanying your loved one to their appointments, if they welcome it, can be incredibly beneficial. This gesture shows your commitment to their well-being and provides you with firsthand insight into their treatment progress and challenges. It also offers an opportunity to ask questions directly to healthcare providers, gaining clarity on how best to support your loved one at home. Sometimes, just being there can make the clinical environment feel less intimidating for your loved one, helping them to communicate more openly with their healthcare provider.

Supporting a loved one in adhering to their treatment plan is what we do, yet can sometimes be challenging. Treatment adherence is not just about reminding them to take their medication or attend therapy sessions; it involves understanding and helping manage the side effects they might be experiencing, which can often be a significant barrier to sticking with treatment. For instance, some antidepressants can cause nausea or sleep disturbances, so being aware of these potential side effects and discussing ways to manage them can help your loved one feel less overwhelmed. Regularly checking in to see how they're feeling about their treatment and if they believe it's helping can also provide encouragement and help you gauge when additional support might be needed.

One of the most uplifting ways to enhance treatment adherence is by celebrating every bit of progress, no matter how small. This could be as simple as acknowledging their effort to stick to their treatment plan or noting improvements in their mood and energy levels. Celebrating these victories can boost their morale, especially on days when they feel they are not making progress. It's important to recognize these moments, as they reinforce the benefits of sticking with treatment and can motivate continued efforts toward recovery.

In supporting someone with SAD, your role is multifaceted but always anchored in empathy, patience, respect, and proactive involvement. By understanding the nuances of SAD treatments, accompanying them to appointments, assisting in managing treatment plans, and celebrating their progress, you provide a foundation of support that can make a significant difference in their treatment journey. This support can help them navigate the challenges of SAD and enhance the strength and resilience of your relationship, providing a shared path toward wellness and recovery.

4.5 PLANNING FOR THE SEASONAL SHIFT: PREEMPTIVE STRATEGIES FOR FAMILIES

When the leaves begin to turn and the air carries a crispness that whispers of the coming winter, families with a loved one affected by Seasonal Affective Disorder (SAD) might feel a twinge of apprehension alongside the beauty of the fall. This period of transition is not just a change in the weather but a herald of the challenges that might resurface with shorter days and longer nights. However, with thoughtful anticipatory planning, families can create a supportive environment that mitigates the impact of SAD and enhances the well-being of everyone involved. This planning involves a proactive adjustment of family routines and an understanding that preparation can transform potential stressors into manageable aspects of daily life.

Creating a supportive environment starts with acknowledging the upcoming seasonal changes and their potential effects openly within the family. More than a family meeting and conversation, it's about actionable steps. This might mean arranging the home environment to maximize light exposure, such as repositioning furniture to sit near windows or ensuring that outdoor spaces are accessible for when the weather still permits. Additionally, investing in light therapy devices before the winter fully sets in can be a practical move. Placing these strategically around the home ensures that your loved one does not have to go out of their way to seek treatment once they start feeling the effects of SAD. It's about integrating these changes seamlessly into the home so that they don't stand as constant reminders of the disorder but are simply part of the environment.

Adjusting family routines is equally valuable. This adjustment means being flexible with commitments and understanding that your loved one's energy levels and mood might fluctuate more dramatically during the winter months. It might be beneficial to discuss as a family how you can shift chores or responsibilities temporarily to accommodate these changes. For instance, if evening activities become too taxing as the season progresses, consider shifting important family activities to earlier in the day or weekend mornings when your loved one might feel more energetic. This shift not only helps in managing the practical aspects of daily life but also ensures that your loved one still feels involved and supported, without the pressure to perform when they are not at their best.

Moreover, adapting family activities to be more SAD-friendly can also involve incorporating more light-filled and engaging activities into your family's routine. This adaptation could mean taking family walks during the early afternoon when the sun is still out or starting a family hobby that can be done in well-lit areas of the home, like crafting or board games. These activities not only help in managing the symptoms of SAD but also strengthen family bonds, creating shared moments that can lift everyone's spirits.

Maintaining open lines of communication is perhaps the pivotal point in all these strategies. Most importantly, that everyone in the family feels comfortable discussing how the changing seasons affect them, without judgment or dismissal. This openness can be fostered through regular family meetings that provide a space for everyone to voice their feelings and concerns about the upcoming winter. It's also a time to collectively brainstorm about ways to support each other, ensuring that the family operates as a cohesive group of individuals living under the same roof, that tackles challenges together.

Lastly, setting flexible expectations, particularly during significant times like the holidays, which can be particularly stressful for someone with SAD. The holidays often come with a set of cultural or familial expectations that may be overwhelming. Discussing and agreeing on what is realistically manageable can alleviate pressure on your loved one and also allow everyone to enjoy the season more fully. This might mean choosing to host fewer guests, opting for simpler meal options, or even creating new traditions that prioritize relaxation and enjoyment over elaborate preparations.

By taking these proactive steps, families can prepare for the seasonal shift with a strategy that supports their loved one with SAD as well as enhance their overall readiness and resilience against the potential challenges of the darker months. These strategies underscore a commitment to flexibility, support, and open communication, which form the foundation by fostering a nurturing family environment where every member feels valued and understood, regardless of the season.

4.6 SELF-CARE FOR CAREGIVERS: MANAGING YOUR OWN WELL-BEING

When you are deeply involved in caring for a loved one with Seasonal Affective Disorder (SAD), it's easy to overlook your own needs. The demands of caregiving can be consuming, leaving little energy for self-reflection or self-care. However, recognizing the signs of caregiver burnout is necessary for maintaining your health and the quality of care you provide. Burnout can manifest in various ways, including persistent tiredness, feelings of despair or irritability, and physical symptoms such as headaches or changes in appetite. You might find yourself feeling unusually detached from your loved one or feeling like your caregiving is never good enough. These signs signal a need to pause and reassess your approach to self-care.

Taking proactive steps towards your own well-being is not selfish; it's necessary. Practical self-care strategies can significantly enhance your resilience. Begin by establishing a routine that includes dedicated time for activities that rejuvenate you. Whether it's a daily walk, reading, yoga, or any activity that you enjoy, make it a non-negotiable part of your day. Nutrition also plays a fundamental role in self-care. Eating balanced meals can help maintain your energy levels and focus, which are essential for effective caregiving. Additionally, ensure you get enough sleep. Sleep deprivation can exacerbate stress, reduce your problem-solving ability, and diminish your capacity for patience—all needed for managing the challenges of caregiving.

Seeking support plays an important role in caregiver self-care. Engaging with caregiver support groups, either in person or online, can provide a valuable outlet for sharing experiences and strategies. These groups offer a sense of community and understanding that can be incredibly comforting. You are reminded that you are not alone in your challenges, and you can learn from the experiences of others who are in similar situations. Therapy or counseling can also be beneficial, providing a space to express and work through the emotional complexities of caregiving. If the demands of caregiving are overwhelming, consider respite care services, which can give you a necessary break to recharge.

Balancing the role of caregiver with other life responsibilities requires thoughtful management of your time and energy. Setting clear boundaries about what you can and cannot do is a good start. Communicate openly with other family members about the need for shared responsibilities, or discuss the possibility of rotating caregiving duties. Learning to delegate where possible, whether within the family or by hiring outside help for certain tasks, can prevent you from taking on too much. Remember, managing your roles effectively isn't about achieving a perfect balance every day but about ongoing adjustments that preserve your well-being over time.

As you navigate the complexities of caring for someone with SAD, remember that your own well-being is a priority. Recognizing signs of burnout, engaging in practical self-care, seeking support, and balancing your roles are all necessary steps to ensure that you can provide care sustainably. By taking care of yourself, you ensure that you have the strength, patience, energy and over all health to care for your loved one, effectively making the journey through the winter months more manageable for you both.

Summarization and Transition to Next Chapter

In this chapter, we've explored the multifaceted role of caregivers in supporting loved ones with Seasonal Affective Disorder, highlighting the importance of communication, understanding treatment options, and proactive crisis management. Most importantly, we've emphasized the vital need for caregivers to prioritize their own well-being. As we move forward, we'll delve into building and leveraging support networks, a fundamental aspect of managing SAD that extends beyond individual efforts to community and societal involvement. This next chapter will guide you in expanding your support strategies, ensuring a robust system that enhances the resilience and well-being of both those affected by SAD and their caregivers.

5

BUILDING AND LEVERAGING SUPPORT NETWORKS

A s the winter sky stretches vast and unyielding above, its stark expanse often mirrors the solitude many feel when grappling with Seasonal Affective Disorder (SAD). Yet, beneath this seemingly endless canopy lies a network, woven with threads of common experiences and shared struggles, offering warmth and strength to those who seek it. This chapter is dedicated to guiding you through the intricate process of finding and integrating into support networks that resonate with your needs and circumstances. Whether these networks are forged online, in the heart of your local community, or even if they spring from your initiative, they hold the potential to significantly alleviate the isolation that SAD can impose.

5.1 FINDING SUPPORT GROUPS: ONLINE AND IN-PERSON RESOURCES

Identifying Resources

In your journey to connect with others who understand the nuances of living with SAD, the first step is identifying where these support networks exist. Both online and in-person resources can offer substantial support, but finding the right one can sometimes feel like searching for a beacon in the fog. Start locally by checking churches, community centers, hospitals, and mental health clinics; many host or can direct you to existing support groups. Libraries and religious institutions often have bulletin boards listing local support meetings. These settings provide a tangible sense of connection, where expressions of empathy are seen in the nods of heads and the sharing of a cup of coffee.

However, the digital landscape has significantly expanded the accessibility of support networks. Online platforms dedicated to mental health, such as Psychology Today or NAMI (National Alliance on Mental Illness), offer directories of support groups that cater specifically to those dealing with SAD. Social media platforms like Facebook and Reddit have communities where thousands share their experiences and strategies for managing SAD. These online groups can be particularly valuable if geographical or physical limitations restrict your access to in-person meetings, or if you prefer the anonymity that online interactions can provide.

Benefits of Support Groups

Engaging with a support group can transform the winter months from a period of dread to one of collective resilience. The primary strength of these groups lies in their ability to dissolve the feeling of isolation by sharing experiences. Hearing others discuss similar struggles and triumphs provides a comforting reassurance that you are not alone. Moreover, these groups often become a well-spring of practical strategies tailored to managing SAD effectively. From tips about the most effective light therapy lamps to recommendations for vitamin supplements or mindfulness exercises, the information shared is both relevant and tested.

These gatherings also serve as a motivational anchor, encouraging consistency in treatment and healthy routines. It's easier to stick to a light therapy schedule or a morning exercise routine when you know others are doing the same and that you'll be sharing your progress. The accountability and mutual encouragement found in support groups can significantly enhance your ability to manage SAD.

Virtual Support Networks

The rise of virtual support networks has been a silver lining, particularly highlighted during times when physical distancing became a norm. These networks offer flexibility that traditional in-person groups might not—such as attending from the comfort of your home and finding meetings that fit your schedule, regardless of time zones. Platforms like Zoom or Google Meet are often used to host virtual meetings, making them accessible to anyone with an internet connection. Moreover, these virtual spaces can connect you with a global community, offering diverse perspectives and remedies that you might not encounter locally.

Starting Your Own Group

Sometimes, the perfect support group is the one you start yourself. If you find that existing groups do not meet your needs or are simply too far away, initiating your own can be a rewarding endeavor. Starting a support group doesn't require you to be an expert on SAD; rather, it's about facilitating a space where people can share and support each other. Utilize online platforms like Meetup for setting up and promoting your group. Local community centers and libraries might also offer space for meetings. Be clear about the group's purpose and who it's for when advertising, and consider setting a structure for meetings to ensure that discussions remain respectful and constructive.

Starting your own group not only fills a gap in your local or online community but also positions you as a proactive member, taking charge of your journey with SAD. It empowers you as you seek support and as you provide it, creating a network that can sustain you and others through the challenges of SAD.

In fostering these connections, whether through finding existing groups or starting your own, you weave a net of shared understanding and mutual support, turning the collective struggle with SAD into a joint quest for well-being and happiness. This chapter serves as your guide in this vital aspect of managing SAD, ensuring that you have the tools and knowledge to find or create a support network that resonates with your needs.

5.2 THE POWER OF PEER SUPPORT: CONNECTING WITH OTHERS WHO UNDERSTAND

In the quiet corners of community centers or the buzzing chat rooms online, there's a unique kind of magic happening—a shared understanding and exchange of stories among individuals who are navigating the complexities of Seasonal Affective Disorder (SAD). This exchange, rooted in peer support, offers more than just mutual commiseration; it's a fertile ground for nurturing resilience and fostering deep connections that can significantly buffer the emotional toll of SAD. When you share your story, it does more than just echo in the ears of listeners; it resonates with their own experiences, creating a bond that can be both affirming and healing.

The act of sharing personal stories within these groups acts as a powerful cathartic experience for many. It's not merely about unburdening oneself or seeking sympathy but about the validation that comes when others nod in understanding, having walked similar paths. This shared narrative can significantly diminish the isolation that so often accompanies SAD, replacing it with a sense of community and shared purpose. Each story contributes to a collective tapestry of experiences, which enriches the support group and enhances each member's understanding of their own journey with SAD. These stories often highlight diverse coping strategies, providing new perspectives and tools that you might not have considered. For instance, hearing how someone successfully managed their symptoms through a combination of light therapy and guided meditation might inspire you to explore similar strategies, broadening your own toolkit for managing SAD.

Peer advice, another cornerstone of support groups, extends beyond conventional wisdom. It's grounded in lived experience, making it uniquely practical and immediately applicable. This advice ranges from the best times to engage in light therapy to how to communicate your needs to those who may not understand the nuances of SAD. Such exchange of advice is often times invaluable; it's tested and tailored to the specific challenges that accompany living with a seasonal disorder. Moreover, this advice often comes with genuine empathy, making it easier to receive and integrate into your own life. The emotional support that accompanies this advice can also be a powerful motivator. Knowing that others are not just surviving but thriving can ignite hope and determination, essential ingredients for managing long-term conditions like SAD.

Building friendships within these groups often evolves naturally. These are not friendships born out of convenience or proximity but out of shared vulnerability and strength. Such connections can provide emotional and social benefits that extend well beyond the structured meetings of a support group. These friendships can become sources of spontaneous joy and comfort, much needed for anyone dealing with the ups and downs of SAD. Whether it's having someone to call on a particularly tough day or celebrating together during periods of remission, these relationships can significantly enhance your quality of life. They create a rich fabric, woven with understanding and mutual support, which stands strong even outside the formal settings of group meetings.

Confidentiality and trust are the pillars on which these peer support groups stand. Safe spaces are cultivated by an agreement to honor each other's stories and struggles without judgment or unsolicited dissemination. This sense of security encourages openness and honesty, which are fundamental for the effectiveness of the support offered. Knowing that the group is a confidential space can make it easier for members to share deeply personal experiences and vulnerabilities, which is where much of the healing and growth occurs. The trust that develops from this confidentiality strengthens the group's dynamic and reinforces each member's commitment to the group and to their own healing process.

In these gatherings, be they virtual or physical, you find more than just companionship; you may discover a mirror reflecting your own struggles and triumphs, a reminder that your experience, though deeply personal, is also part of a larger narrative. This realization can be profoundly comforting and empowering, providing you with the strength to face the darker days with the knowledge that you are not alone, and more importantly, that there is a community that understands and stands with you.

5.3 COMMUNICATING YOUR NEEDS: STRATEGIES FOR SAD SUFFERERS

Living with Seasonal Affective Disorder (SAD) can sometimes feel like navigating a complex labyrinth of emotions and misunderstandings, especially when trying to communicate your needs to those around you. Assertive communication is a skill that, when honed, can significantly improve how effectively you express your needs, wants, limits and boundaries, ensuring they are understood and respected by family, friends, and coworkers. Being assertive involves expressing your thoughts and feelings openly and honestly while maintaining respect for the other person. This might mean saying something like, "I appreciate your invitation to go out tonight, but I'm feeling quite drained and need some time to rest due to my SAD. Can we reschedule for another day?" This kind of communication not only conveys your needs clearly but also invites understanding and respect for your condition, reducing potential feelings of guilt or misunderstanding.

Setting healthy boundaries is another determinant aspect of managing interactions when you have SAD. It's about understanding your limits and communicating these to the people in your life. For example, if long evening social engagements exacerbate your symptoms, you might set a boundary by limiting such activities or ensuring there's a quiet space available if you need a break. Communicating these boundaries clearly and preemptively can help manage expectations and prevent situations that might lead to stress or discomfort. It's helpful to explain why these boundaries are necessary, perhaps by sharing how certain situations affect your symptoms, as this can help others understand the rationale behind your needs, fostering greater empathy and cooperation. It's a delicate balance between how much information is too much vs just enough.

Asking for help is often impeded by barriers such as pride or the fear of being a burden. These feelings are common, but overcoming them is essential for managing SAD effectively. Start by acknowledging that seeking help is a sign of strength, not weakness. It shows a commitment to managing your health and maintaining your relationships. When asking for help, be specific about what you need, whether it's assistance in daily tasks during particularly tough times or just the company of a friend when you're feeling low. Remember, most loved ones will appreciate the opportunity to provide support; it helps them feel engaged and useful, strengthening the bond between you.

Navigating misunderstandings or dismissive attitudes towards SAD involves a proactive approach to education and dialogue. Misconceptions about SAD can lead to comments or behaviors from others that may seem minimizing or insensitive. Addressing these requires a calm and informed response. For instance, if someone remarks that everyone gets the winter blues and you should just "snap out of it," consider this an opportunity to educate them about SAD. You might explain that while many people might feel down during shorter days, SAD is a recognized medical condition that can significantly impact one's life. If they are receptive, sharing articles, videos, or other educational materials can also help others understand your experience more deeply. Furthermore, suggesting them to join discussions or support groups can provide them a broader perspective on the condition, potentially transforming their understanding and approach towards you and your shared experiences. There are also those individuals who are set in their limited knowledge and have no desire to learn otherwise. Not to be taken personally as that is where they are in their human journey, yet you might consider investing your time and energy with individuals that correlate with your own intrinsic values. Thus demonstrating a broader concept of 'limits and boundaries'.

By mastering assertive communication, setting clear boundaries, asking for help confidently, and effectively handling misunderstandings, you empower yourself to navigate the challenges of SAD with greater ease and support. These strategies enhance your ability to cope with SAD and potentially enrich your interactions and relationships, creating a more supportive and understanding environment around you. As you continue to advocate for your needs and educate those around you, remember that each conversation is a step toward broader awareness and acceptance, not just for you but for the many others who live with SAD.

5.4 LEVERAGING SOCIAL MEDIA FOR SUPPORT AND AWARENESS

In today's digitally connected world, social media platforms have transcended their initial purpose of mere social networking, morphing into vital tools for information dissemination, community building, and advocacy. For individuals grappling with Seasonal Affective Disorder (SAD), these platforms offer unique avenues to seek support, share experiences, and raise awareness about this often-misunderstood condition. However, the key to harnessing the full potential of social media lies in its positive and strategic use. By crafting an approach that emphasizes connection and education while navigating the inherent pitfalls of online interactions, you can create a supportive online environment that extends well beyond your immediate geographical boundaries.

The first step in utilizing social media positively is to curate your feeds and interactions to foster a supportive network. This means following reputable mental health organizations, joining groups or pages dedicated to SAD, and connecting with individuals who share constructive content. Platforms like Instagram and Facebook allow you to follow hashtags such as #SADsupport or #MentalHealthAwareness, which can lead you to valuable content and communities. Engage actively but thoughtfully with these communities by sharing your experiences and insights, asking questions, and offering support to others. This active engagement helps in building a network that is supportive, enriches your understanding of SAD as well as various coping strategies.

However, the world of social media is not without potential pitfalls, such as the propensity for comparison or the exposure to negative interactions. To navigate these challenges, it is advisable to set clear boundaries for your social media use. Limit your time spent on platforms to avoid overload and consider using features that allow you to control what you see in your feed, such as muting or unfollowing accounts that trigger negative feelings or contribute to a sense of inadequacy. Remember, the goal is to make your social media experience empowering and supportive, not draining or distressing.

Social media also serves as a powerful platform for awareness campaigns about SAD. By sharing personal stories and educational content, you can shed light on the realities of living with SAD, helping to dispel myths and reduce stigma. Consider creating or sharing posts that describe what SAD is, detailing symptoms, and emphasizing the difference between SAD and general winter blues. Infographics, short videos, and even interactive stories can capture the attention of a wide audience, spreading knowledge and fostering a better understanding of SAD. You might also share updates from your own life about managing SAD, such as your daily routine during the winter months, how you use light therapy, or the impact of diet and exercise on your well-being. These personal insights provide a relatable and humanized perspective on managing SAD, making the condition more accessible and comprehensible to those unfamiliar with it.

Finding and engaging with online communities dedicated to SAD and mental health support can further enhance your social media experience. These communities offer a platform to connect with individuals who can relate to your experiences, providing opportunities for mutual support. Look for groups that have active moderation and clear guidelines to ensure discussions remain respectful and supportive. Participate in scheduled live sessions, webinars, or online workshops that many of these communities offer, which can provide additional learning opportunities and a sense of real-time connection with others.

Finally, consider the importance of privacy when sharing personal experiences or seeking support on social media platforms. While openness can be therapeutic and beneficial in raising awareness, it's important to consider how much personal information you share online. Utilize privacy settings offered by social media platforms to control who can see your posts. Be cautious about sharing details that could compromise your or anyone else's privacy. Engaging anonymously in specific forums can sometimes offer a way to seek support while protecting your identity, particularly if you are discussing sensitive issues.

By leveraging social media effectively, you enhance your own support system and contribute to a broader awareness and understanding of SAD. This thoughtful engagement transforms your social media platforms from mere communication tools into active components of your wellness strategy, where connections, learning, and personal growth go hand in hand.

5.5 NURTURING RELATIONSHIPS DESPITE SEASONAL CHALLENGES

Navigating relationships during periods of Seasonal Affective Disorder (SAD) presents a unique set of challenges. The fluctuating nature of SAD means that during certain times of the year, individuals might find their mood, energy levels, and general outlook significantly altered, which can strain personal interactions. Recognizing the need for both understanding and patience is foundational during these times. It is essential for those around someone experiencing SAD to appreciate that this condition does not just affect mood, it can alter the person's capacity to engage in social activities, communicate effectively, or show affection in conventional ways. Patience becomes a necessity, not just an advantage. It helps in giving the person with SAD the space to manage their symptoms without feeling pressured to 'snap out of it' – a common misconception about managing mood disorders. Moreover, understanding that this condition is cyclical can prepare both parties to anticipate and plan for tougher periods, reducing potential frustrations that arise from unmet expectations.

In relationships, open and honest communication is always touted as key, but for those experiencing low periods due to SAD, it becomes even more significant. Keeping communication channels open during these times ensures that misunderstandings are minimized and that both parties feel supported and connected. It's about expressing what you feel and what you might need—be it space, a listening ear, or just the presence of someone who cares—

without the fear of judgment. For the partner or family members without SAD, initiating gentle conversations about how the condition might be influencing their loved one's behavior or feelings can be insightful. This openness allows for a shared understanding and collaborative management of the condition, reinforcing the relationship's foundation during potentially turbulent times.

Balancing the dynamics of support and independence in any relationship where chronic conditions like SAD are involved can be delicate. On one hand, the desire to be supportive might lead one to overextend, hovering over the person with SAD, potentially leading to feelings of suffocation or loss of autonomy. On the other hand, too much detachment can make the person with SAD feel neglected or abandoned. Striking a balance involves recognizing and respecting the individual's need for independence while still providing an adequate level of support. This balance can be negotiated and adjusted through ongoing dialogue, ensuring that both parties feel comfortable with the level of interdependence. Encouraging activities that foster independence for the person with SAD, such as pursuing hobbies or social interactions outside the home, can also be beneficial. These activities can provide a sense of control and normalcy, important for mental health and the overall dynamism of the relationship.

Considering couples or family therapy is another beneficial strategy for addressing the complexities SAD introduces into relationships. Therapy provides a structured environment where both parties can express their feelings, fears, and frustrations safely and constructively. It's an opportunity to explore how SAD affects their relationship under the guidance of a professional who can offer practical strategies tailored to their specific situation. This therapeutic setting can foster mutual understanding and growth, helping both parties navigate the challenges of SAD with greater empathy and cooperation. Therapists can also help identify patterns that may exacerbate the condition or the relationship dynamics, offering insights that are often harder to self-identify. This professional guidance can be instrumental in transforming potential relationship pitfalls into strengthening moments, ultimately allowing the relationship to thrive despite the seasonal challenges brought by SAD.

In every interaction within these dynamics, the emphasis on mutual respect, understanding, and patience guides each party through the seasonal highs and lows. This approach maintains the relationship's health and supports the personal growth of both individuals. Whether it's through enhanced communication, a thoughtful balance of support and independence, or professional guidance, the aim is to ensure that the relationship not only survives but also becomes a reliable source of comfort and strength throughout the changing seasons.

5.6 PROFESSIONAL HELP: WHEN AND HOW TO SEEK IT

Navigating the waters of Seasonal Affective Disorder (SAD) often requires more than just the warm handholds of family and friends or the shared experiences within support groups. There comes a point where professional help might become necessary to effectively manage the more challenging aspects of SAD. Recognizing when to seek this help can be challenging; it hinges on observing certain signs that indicate your current strategies may no longer be sufficient. These signs might include persistent feelings of sadness or hopelessness that don't improve despite using light therapy, lifestyle changes, or basic counseling. You might also experience severe changes in sleep patterns, appetite, or energy levels, or find that your symptoms are beginning to significantly interfere with your daily responsibilities and relationships. When these signs begin to echo loudly in your daily life, it's a clear signal that seeking professional help could provide the additional support you need.

Finding the right mental health professional is the next step once you decide to seek help. This process can feel daunting, but knowing what to look for can simplify it. Ideally, you want to find a professional who has experience with SAD. Psychiatrists, psychologists, and licensed therapists with a background in treating mood disorders can offer more specialized care. Start by consulting your primary care provider, who can provide a referral. Alternatively, use reputable sources like the American Psychological Association's psychologist locator to find a suitable professional. When selecting a therapist or psychiatrist, it's important to consider their treatment approach and ensure it aligns with your preferences. For instance, you might prefer cognitive-behavioral therapy because of its structured approach to solving problems, or you might be more inclined towards a therapist who integrates holistic practices like mindfulness in their treatment regimen.

Integrating professional support with your existing support networks is essential for a comprehensive approach to managing SAD. Effective integration means that all parties—your healthcare provider, family, friends, and any support groups you belong to— are informed of each other's roles and are working collaboratively towards your wellness. This might involve family therapy sessions where your loved ones learn about SAD directly from a professional, or it could be as simple as your therapist and your primary care doctor exchanging information about your treatment progress and any medications prescribed. This holistic approach ensures that every angle of your SAD management is being addressed, which can significantly improve your overall treatment outcome.

Addressing concerns about insurance coverage and accessibility is also an impactful part of seeking professional help. Mental health services can be expensive, but many insurance plans do cover psychological counseling and psychiatric treatment, often requiring just a co-pay. Before you schedule an appointment, check with your insurance provider to understand what services are covered and if you need a referral from your primary care physician to see a specialist. If insurance coverage is inadequate or non-existent, look for community health centers or university psychology departments, which often offer counseling services at a reduced cost. These services are typically provided by supervised students and can be an excellent, affordable option for receiving support.

Navigating the decision to seek professional help can often feel like an uphill journey, but recognizing the need, finding the right professional, integrating their support, and addressing insurance and accessibility concerns can equip you with a robust plan for managing SAD. These steps can enhance your ability to cope with the disorder and empower you to take proactive steps toward your mental health and well-being.

In wrapping up this chapter, we've traversed the essential avenues for building and leveraging your support networks, from the grassroots of community and online support groups to the structured care provided by health professionals. Each layer of support offers unique benefits and, when woven together, they form a comprehensive safety net that sustains you through the winter months. As we turn our focus in the next chapter to the broader societal understanding and treatment of SAD, remember that the journey toward managing this condition is not walked alone. The networks you build, the professionals you engage, and the personal strategies you implement all play integral roles in navigating Seasonal Affective Disorder effectively.

BEYOND THE BASICS

6.1 SAD IN THE WORKPLACE: RIGHTS, RESPONSIBILITIES, AND STRATEGIES

As the winter months unfold, bringing shorter days and less sunlight, many individuals find themselves grappling with more than just the cold weather. For those experiencing Seasonal Affective Disorder (SAD), these months can significantly impact their professional lives, manifesting challenges that extend beyond personal health and into their work environment. Understanding your rights and the responsibilities of your employer can empower you to advocate for a workspace that prioritizes and actively supports your well-being.

Understanding Worker Rights

Under various disability rights laws, such as the Americans with Disabilities Act (ADA) in the United States, employees suffering from SAD may be entitled to reasonable accommodations, provided they have a documented condition that substantially limits one or more major life activities. This recognition classifies SAD not merely as a seasonal inconvenience but as a medical condition that can affect your ability to perform job functions effectively. As such, you are entitled to request accommodations that might alleviate these difficulties. These accommodations could range from a workspace with more natural light to flexible work hours that allow for exposure to daylight. It's important to note that while employers are required to provide accommodations, these must not impose an undue hardship on the operation of the business. Understanding these rights, arms you with the knowledge necessary to initiate conversations about your needs, and sets a legal framework that supports these discussions.

Employer Responsibilities

For employers, the challenge often lies not in the refusal to accommodate but in recognizing the need for such accommodations. Employers are responsible for providing a work environment that does not discriminate against those with disabilities, including seasonal affective disorder. This responsibility includes recognizing the legitimacy of SAD as a medical condition, which requires an informed understanding of its symptoms and impacts. Employers should foster an environment where employees feel comfortable disclosing their conditions without fear of stigma or repercussions—a vital step in managing workplace health and productivity. Training sessions that educate managers and HR professionals about SAD and other mental health issues can be an integral part of developing this supportive work culture.

Effective Workplace Strategies

Beyond legal accommodations, there are practical strategies that can be implemented to ease the burden of SAD on affected employees. Light therapy, one of the most effective treatments for SAD, can be incorporated into the workplace by providing light therapy lamps in common areas or allowing employees to have them at their desks. Flexibility in work hours can also be a significant aid; for instance, allowing employees to come in later during the winter months and make up the hours at times when it's still daylight can make a substantial difference in their mental health and productivity. Remote work options, which have become more feasible due to technological advancements, can also be considered to allow employees to manage their environment according to their needs.

Advocacy and Awareness

Fostering workplace initiatives that promote awareness about SAD can transform an office environment into a supportive space that recognizes and actively combats the challenges faced with this disorder. Initiatives could include workshops led by mental health professionals, distribution of informative materials, or even peer-led sessions where employees share strategies that have personally helped them manage SAD. Such efforts educate the workforce and contribute to destigmatizing the condition, making it easier for employees to seek help and accommodations. Moreover, these initiatives can encourage a culture of openness and proactive care, which can significantly enhance overall employee well-being and cohesion.

In navigating SAD in the workplace, the convergence of legal knowledge, supportive employer practices, personal advocacy, and broad awareness creates a holistic approach that addresses the immediate needs of those affected and also fosters a broader cultural shift towards inclusive and health-conscious work environments. This shift is essential for enhancing productivity. By nurturing a work culture that values and supports the well-being of every employee, it reinforces a healthy workforce that is inherently more vibrant, engaged, and resilient.

Interactive Element: Reflection Section

Consider reflecting on your current work environment in relation to your experience with SAD:

- How does your workplace acknowledge or accommodate mental health needs?
- What accommodations do you think would help you manage your symptoms effectively during work hours?
- How comfortable do you feel discussing SAD with your employer or colleagues?

Engaging with these questions can help you assess the current support structures at your workplace and identify areas for advocacy and improvement. This reflection process can aid in personalizing your approach to managing SAD at work and contribute to ongoing dialogues about mental health in professional settings. Ultimately, fostering a more inclusive and supportive work culture.

6.2 SEASONAL AFFECTIVE DISORDER IN CHILDREN AND ADOLESCENTS

When we consider Seasonal Affective Disorder (SAD), our thoughts often turn immediately to adults battling the dreary mood swings brought on by shorter days and longer nights. Yet, it's important to recognize that children and adolescents are not immune to this seasonal challenge. The manifestation of SAD in young people can sometimes be more subtle or mistaken for other behavioral issues, which makes discerning its symptoms all the more impactful. Typically, children and teenagers with SAD might exhibit irritability, a noticeable decline in interest in activities they usually enjoy, or a pervasive sense of lethargy that goes beyond normal tiredness. Unlike adults, who might articulate feelings of sadness or hopelessness, young people are more likely to demonstrate behavioral changes such as trouble concentrating on schoolwork, withdrawal from social interactions, or increased sensitivity to rejection.

The ripple effects of SAD in the lives of young individuals extend into their educational and social spheres significantly. Academically, the decreased concentration and energy can lead to a noticeable decline in performance, which is often misinterpreted as a lack of effort or motivation. Socially, the withdrawal and irritability attributable to SAD can strain friendships, leaving peers puzzled by the sudden change in demeanor. This withdrawal can exacerbate feelings of isolation, feeding into a cycle that can further deepen depressive symptoms. The impact is profound; it touches on the foundational aspects of a young person's life that are essential for their development and overall well-being.

Addressing SAD in children and adolescents requires a proactive approach from both parents and educators. Parents can support their children by maintaining a routine that maximizes exposure to natural light, such as ensuring that curtains are open during the day or encouraging outdoor activities during daylight hours. It's also beneficial to maintain a dialogue about mood and feelings, providing a safe space for children to express themselves without fear of judgment. This open line of communication can help parents gauge their child's emotional state and better understand when to seek further support if needed.

Educators also play a pivotal role, as they are in a unique position to notice changes in a student's behavior or academic performance that may be indicative of SAD. Schools can implement strategies such as ensuring classrooms receive ample natural light or scheduling outdoor activities during school hours to combat the effects of limited daylight exposure. Moreover, teacher training on mental health issues can be invaluable, equipping educators with the knowledge to recognize signs of SAD and the competence to approach the subject sensitively with both the student and their parents.

In terms of treatment, the options for children and adolescents largely mirror those for adults, yet they must be approached with careful consideration of the young person's age and developmental stage. Light therapy can be effective; however, it requires supervision to ensure it is used safely. Psychotherapy, particularly Cognitive Behavioral Therapy (CBT), tailored to younger age groups, can help children develop coping strategies to manage their symptoms. In some cases, medication may be considered, but this is generally pursued only after other treatments have been tried and under careful medical supervision, given the different impacts and side effects drugs may have on young bodies and minds.

Early intervention is paramount. By addressing SAD when symptoms first appear, parents and educators can help mitigate the more severe impacts of the disorder. This proactive approach aids in managing the immediate symptoms and contributes to the long-term mental health and academic success of the child. Engaging with these strategies transforms the challenging months of SAD into a manageable period, ensuring that children and adolescents have the support and tools they need to not only cope, but thrive despite the seasonal challenges they face.

6.3 THE GEOGRAPHY OF SAD: HOW LOCATION INFLUENCES SYMPTOMS

The prevalence and intensity of Seasonal Affective Disorder (SAD) can significantly depend on geographical factors, most notably the latitude of your location. The further you live from the equator, the more likely you are to experience the reduced sunlight exposure that often triggers the symptoms of SAD. This relationship between latitude and SAD is not just a matter of shorter days; it's also about the quality of light during those days, which can be much dimmer and less intense in the northern or southern extremities of the globe. This reduced intensity affects the body's circadian rhythms and can disrupt the natural production of melatonin and serotonin, critical regulators of sleep and mood. For instance, residents of Norway or Alaska may find themselves particularly susceptible to these disruptions due to their extreme latitudinal positions, which result in very short days during the winter months.

Beyond latitude, local climate patterns play a big role in the manifestation of SAD. Areas characterized by prolonged periods of cloudiness or rain, such as the Pacific Northwest of the United States or much of the United Kingdom, can exacerbate the challenges of limited sunlight. Even if these regions do not necessarily boast extreme latitudinal coordinates, the persistent overcast conditions can mimic the effects of shorter winter days, limiting exposure to precious sunlight. This lack of light can prolong or intensify the depressive episodes associated with SAD, making it imperative for residents in these climates to seek alternative sources of light or treatment methods to diminish the effects.

Considering relocation as a strategy to manage SAD is a significant decision that comes with its own set of challenges and considerations. While moving to a location with more favorable winter light conditions might seem like an ideal solution, it's important to weigh this against the practical implications such as the impact on social ties, employment, and general lifestyle. For those for whom relocation is a feasible option, it might indeed offer a substantial improvement in managing SAD symptoms. However, it's diligent to approach such a decision with comprehensive planning and consultation with medical professionals to ensure that the benefits outweigh the potential stresses or disruptions that significant relocation might entail.

For many, however, relocation is not a practical solution. In such cases, adapting to the environment becomes essential. Maximizing light exposure wherever possible can significantly help manage SAD symptoms. This adaptation might involve structuring indoor living and working spaces to enhance light intake, such as positioning desks near windows or using mirrors to reflect natural light more effectively within a room. Additionally, making a conscious effort to spend time outdoors during daylight hours, even when sunlight seems minimal, can help in maintaining a healthier circadian rhythm. For those in particularly challenging climates, artificial light sources such as light therapy lamps can be invaluable. These lamps are designed to mimic natural sunlight and can be used to provide therapeutic benefits, especially when used during the morning hours to simulate dawn and reduce the overproduction of melatonin.

In understanding the geographical influences on SAD, it becomes clear that while the disorder can present significant challenges, there are numerous strategies, both natural and artificial, that can help reduce its impact. Whether through relocation, strategic use of light, or simply adapting lifestyle choices to maximize exposure to available natural light, individuals affected by SAD can find effective ways to manage their symptoms and improve their quality of life during the darker months. The key is in recognizing the specific challenges posed by one's environment and responding with intentional, informed actions that align with personal circumstances and medical guidance.

6.4 SAD THROUGH THE AGES: MANAGING AT ANY STAGE OF LIFE

Seasonal Affective Disorder (SAD) does not discriminate by age; it traverses the spectrum from the vibrancy of youth to the wisdom of older years, each stage bringing its unique set of challenges and strategies for management. Understanding how SAD impacts different life stages allows for a more tailored and effective approach to treatment, ensuring that each individual, regardless of age, can find relief and maintain a quality of life that resonates with their personal journey.

Lifecycle Approach

The manifestation of SAD in an individual's life can vary significantly with age. Adolescents might experience SAD with an irritable mood and a noticeable decline in school performance, which could easily be mistaken for typical teenage behavior or academic disinterest. Adults may face challenges in balancing work responsibilities and personal life while battling the energy dips and mood swings brought on by SAD. In older adults, symptoms might be misattributed to age-related changes or other health conditions, leading to underdiagnosis or misdiagnosis. Recognizing the nuances of how SAD presents at different life stages is necessary for effective identification and management. This nuanced approach ensures that interventions are not only timely but also appropriate, considering the physical, emotional, and social developmental stages of the individual affected.

Age-Specific Strategies

Tailoring strategies to effectively manage SAD involves considering the lifestyle, health status, and social environments typical of
each age group. For younger individuals, integrating light therapy
sessions during morning routines can be beneficial, especially
when combined with engaging physical activities that can boost
overall energy levels and mood. Parents and educators can support
by ensuring environments are well-lit and encouraging outdoor
activities during daylight hours, weather permitting. For working
adults, negotiating flexible work hours to maximize daylight exposure or creating a workplace environment with ample natural light
can be effective strategies. Employers can support this by fostering
a workplace culture that recognizes and adapts to mental health
needs, ensuring that employees do not feel penalized for experiencing seasonal mood variations. In the case of older adults,
ensuring that living spaces are equipped with adequate lighting
becomes essential, alongside regular social interactions to combat
the isolation that can exacerbate SAD symptoms. Healthcare
providers can assist by being vigilant about screening for SAD
during routine health visits, particularly in patients who report a
seasonal pattern in mood changes.

Generational Perspectives on Mental Health

The understanding and acceptance of mental health issues,
including SAD, can vary widely between generations. Older generations might have grown up at a time when mental health was not
as openly discussed, possibly leading to hesitancy in acknowledging or seeking help for symptoms of SAD. In contrast, younger
generations are typically more aware and accepting of mental
health discussions, potentially leading to earlier recognition and
treatment of SAD. Bridging these generational gaps in under-

standing and approach can involve open family discussions about mental health, where experiences and perspectives are shared and validated. Educational programs targeting various age groups can also play a significant role in normalizing mental health care and encouraging a more proactive approach to managing conditions like SAD.

Eldercare and SAD

Elderly individuals often face a unique set of challenges when it comes to managing SAD. Age-related changes such as retirement, the loss of loved ones, decreased mobility, and other health issues can compound the effects of SAD, making management increasingly complex. Recognizing signs of SAD in the elderly is fundamental, as symptoms such as withdrawal from social activities, loss of interest in hobbies, or changes in sleep patterns can significantly impact their overall health and quality of life. Strategies to assist might include ensuring that their living environments are well-lit and that they have regular, structured daily activities that promote social interaction and physical activity. Regular medical check-ups should include assessments for signs of depression and SAD, with treatments adjusted for any existing medical conditions or comorbidities that are prevalent in the elderly.

In addressing SAD across different life stages, the approach must be as dynamic and adaptable as the individuals it aims to support. By acknowledging the specific needs and challenges inherent to each stage of life, strategies can be tailored to manage the symptoms of SAD effectively and enhance the overall well-being of those affected, ensuring that each season of life can be navigated with resilience and support.

6.5 CULTURAL PERSPECTIVES ON SAD AND MENTAL HEALTH

When exploring the multifaceted landscape of Seasonal Affective Disorder (SAD), it becomes evident that cultural perspectives play a significant role in how symptoms are recognized, understood, and treated across different societies. The cultural stigma associated with mental health issues can vary dramatically from one region to another, deeply influencing individuals' willingness to seek help. In some cultures, mental health issues like SAD might be stigmatized to the extent that individuals feel compelled to hide their struggles rather than seeking treatment. This stigma often stems from traditional beliefs about mental health that equate such conditions with personal weakness or a lack of spiritual discipline. Overcoming these cultural barriers requires targeted education and outreach programs that respect cultural nuances while promoting an understanding of SAD as a medical condition that benefits from professional intervention.

The contrast between traditional and Western medicine approaches to treating SAD also highlights significant cultural dynamics. In many Eastern cultures, traditional practices such as herbal medicine, acupuncture, mindfulness practices, mediation, Reiki, Yoga, Tai Chi, and specific dietary adjustments are commonly employed to alleviate symptoms of depression and mood disorders linked to seasonal changes. These methods are often based on holistic principles that consider physical, emotional, and spiritual health inseparably linked. While Western medicine typically focuses on symptom management through pharmacology and psychotherapy, including light therapy specifically for SAD, integrating these diverse approaches can provide more comprehensive treatment options. For instance, individuals might find combining light therapy with mindfulness practices, yoga and herbal supplements that promote serotonin production offers a more effective way to manage their symptoms. This integration requires open-mindedness and respect from healthcare providers for different cultural practices and beliefs about health and wellness.

Building effective cross-cultural support systems for individuals suffering from SAD involves acknowledging and integrating these diverse cultural perspectives into treatment and support strategies. It is imperative for mental health professionals to develop cultural competence, which includes understanding the cultural background of their patients and the different stigmas and health beliefs that influence their perceptions and acceptance of SAD. For example, in communities where discussing mental health is taboo, anonymous support groups or online forums might provide essential support mechanisms that respect cultural sensitivities. Moreover, community leaders and respected figures can play a dynamic role in changing perceptions by speaking openly about mental health, thus gradually reducing stigma and encouraging more individuals to seek help.

Global research on SAD offers a broader perspective on how this disorder is experienced and treated worldwide, revealing both universal challenges and unique cultural responses. Studies indicate that while the prevalence of SAD in countries with long, dark winters is expectedly high, the disorder also affects populations in sunnier climates, albeit differently. These insights challenge the assumption that SAD is solely a product of environmental factors, suggesting that genetic predispositions, lifestyle, and social factors also play significant roles. Such research underscores the importance of a global dialogue in mental health that leverages diverse cultural insights to foster more effective and culturally sensitive approaches to managing SAD. Sharing global research and case studies can help demystify SAD and encourage a more proactive, inclusive approach to diagnosis and treatment across different cultural contexts.

In understanding and addressing SAD, it is clear that cultural perspectives significantly shape the experiences of those affected. By embracing a more culturally inclusive approach, healthcare providers can ensure that all individuals, regardless of their cultural background, have access to supportive and effective treatment options. This approach enhances individual outcomes and contributes to a more holistic understanding of SAD, enriching the collective knowledge and strategies employed to manage this complex disorder. Through continued education, research, and respectful integration of diverse cultural practices, the path to managing SAD can become more accessible and effective for everyone, no matter where they live or what cultural beliefs they hold.

6.6 TECHNOLOGY USE AND SAD: THE PROS AND CONS

In our increasingly digital world, technology plays a multifaceted role in managing Seasonal Affective Disorder (SAD), offering both innovative solutions and posing unique challenges. One of the more significant advancements in this area is the development of digital light solutions, such as light therapy apps and blue light screens, designed to mitigate the symptoms of SAD by simulating natural sunlight. These digital solutions are particularly valuable for individuals who may not have easy access to natural light during the shorter days of winter months. Light therapy apps, for example, can be used on personal devices, providing users with a portable and convenient source of light that mimics the spectrum of natural sunlight. Similarly, blue light screens installed on various devices can help regulate the body's circadian rhythms, which are often disrupted by the lack of sunlight in winter, thus improving mood and sleep patterns.

However, while these technologies offer significant benefits, they also come with drawbacks. The efficacy of these digital solutions can vary widely, and they often do not provide the same level of light intensity as a dedicated light therapy box, which can deliver up to 10,000 lux of light. Users might find that while these apps and devices offer a temporary boost, they may not be sufficient for those with more severe manifestations of SAD. Additionally, the use of these technologies, particularly around bedtime, can interfere with natural sleep patterns, potentially countering some of the benefits by disrupting the body's production of melatonin.

Turning to the realm of social media, its role in the lives of those with SAD is paradoxical. On one hand, platforms like Facebook, Twitter, and Instagram can provide vital social connections that help mitigate feelings of isolation, a common symptom of SAD. These platforms allow individuals to maintain relationships and support networks without needing to leave the comfort of their home, which can be particularly appealing during a depressive episode. Moreover, social media can serve as a powerful tool for raising awareness about SAD, offering platforms where individuals can share experiences, advice, and support.

On the other hand, excessive use of social media has been linked to increased feelings of depression and anxiety, which can exacerbate the symptoms of SAD. The curated portrayals of life that dominate these platforms can lead to detrimental comparisons and a sense of inadequacy, which can further spiral into depressive symptoms. Therefore, while social media holds potential as a supportive resource, it is important for users to be mindful of their consumption habits and the impact these platforms have on their mental health.

The advent of online support resources and therapy options has significantly transformed the landscape of mental health support, making it more accessible to those who might otherwise struggle to find help. Online therapy platforms, for instance, offer sessions with licensed therapists via video calls, chats, or phone calls, providing flexibility and privacy that can be particularly appealing for someone dealing with SAD. These platforms often extend beyond traditional therapy hours, offering late-night or early-morning sessions that can accommodate various schedules and symptoms patterns. Furthermore, numerous websites and forums dedicated to mental health allow individuals to seek information, share their experiences, and connect with others experiencing similar challenges, fostering a virtual community of support.

Mindfulness and meditation apps also offer valuable tools for managing SAD. These apps provide guided sessions that can help users reduce stress, manage anxiety, and improve mood, which are foundational for combating the symptoms of SAD. The portability of these apps allows users to engage in mindfulness exercises at their convenience, perhaps during a lunch break or in the tranquility of their living room. This accessibility makes it easier to incorporate mindfulness into daily routines, providing a consistent tool that can help stabilize mood throughout the winter months.

In sum, while technology offers innovative tools and broadened access to support for managing SAD, it also requires careful consideration and management to ensure these tools are used effectively and do not inadvertently worsen symptoms. As we continue to integrate technology into mental health management, it is diligent to balance these modern conveniences with mindful usage and an awareness of the potential psychological impacts.

Brief Ending to the Chapter

This exploration of technology's role in managing Seasonal Affective Disorder highlights a landscape where innovation meets tradition, offering new tools and challenges. From digital light solutions that bring sunshine into our pockets to the dual-edged sword of social media, the digital age presents novel opportunities and considerations for those battling SAD. As we harness these technological advancements, maintaining a balance between digital and real-world interactions will be defining. Moving forward, the next chapter will delve deeper into the personal narratives of those who navigate life with SAD, providing insights into the diverse ways individuals cope with and overcome the challenges of this seasonal disorder.

7

INTEGRATIVE AND HOLISTIC APPROACHES

As the chill of winter sets in, and the light of day shortens, those grappling with Seasonal Affective Disorder (SAD) often find themselves seeking refuge not just from the cold, but from the shadow it casts over their mood and energy levels. It is here, in the quiet introspection that winter often invites, that holistic approaches such as yoga emerge as beacons of warmth and healing. Yoga, an ancient practice rooted in creating harmony between mind and body, offers more than just physical benefits; it is a holistic therapy that nurtures the mental and emotional resilience necessary to navigate the complexities of SAD.

7.1 YOGA AND SAD: PRACTICES FOR MIND AND BODY HARMONY

The integration of yoga into the management of SAD is grounded in its ability to enhance physical wellness while simultaneously fostering mental clarity and emotional stability. The holistic nature of yoga lies in its combination of physical postures (asana), controlled breathing (pranayama), and meditation, all of which converge to rebalance the body's responses to stress and mood alterations associated with SAD. The practice of yoga stimulates the parasympathetic nervous system — the body's rest and digest system — which can help quell the fight-or-flight response often heightened in anxiety and depression. This type of stimulation is needed for those experiencing SAD, as it encourages a state of relaxation and rejuvenation, countering the lethargy and sadness typical of the disorder.

Specific Yoga Poses for SAD

Yoga offers a variety of poses that can specifically target the symptoms of SAD. For beginners or those seasoned in yoga, certain asanas are particularly beneficial. For instance, backbends like Cobra Pose (Bhujangasana) or Bridge Pose (Setu Bandhasana) are excellent for opening the chest, enhancing breath capacity, and invigorating the body and mind. These poses counteract the common tendency to hunch or close off during depressive episodes, promoting an open, expansive posture that can lead to improved mood and energy levels. Forward bends such as Child's Pose (Balasana) and Seated Forward Bend (Paschimottanasana) are known for their calming effects on the brain and nervous system, making them beneficial for those moments when you need to foster inner peace and relaxation.

Breathwork for Emotional Regulation

Pranayama, or breath control practices, form another cornerstone of yoga that is particularly effective in managing the emotional and psychological aspects of SAD. Techniques such as Nadi Shodhana (Alternate Nostril Breathing) are known for their ability to balance the body's energy channels and harmonize the left and right hemispheres of the brain, enhancing emotional equilibrium and mental clarity. Similarly, the practice of Bhramari Pranayama (Bee Breath) can be immensely soothing for the mind, reducing stress and anxiety by generating a meditative state through the soothing sound of the humming breath.

Incorporating Yoga into Daily Routine

Integrating yoga into your daily routine need not be a daunting task. It can be as simple as dedicating a few minutes each morning to perform a series of sun salutations or engaging in a brief session of breath-focused meditation before bed. The key is consistency and mindfulness; even a few moments of yoga can significantly impact your mood and outlook, providing a sense of control and peace that can help navigate the challenges of SAD. For those new to yoga, many online platforms and local studios offer classes specifically designed for mental health, providing guided, gentle introductions to the practice. Additionally, many yoga apps and YouTube channels offer free sessions that can be done at home, making this practice accessible to all.

Yoga, with its rich tradition of promoting physical, mental, and spiritual wellness, offers a powerful tool for those battling the winter blues associated with SAD. Its ability to integrate body movement, breath control, and meditation creates a comprehensive therapeutic modality that alleviates the physical symptoms of SAD and cultivates the mental resilience necessary to embrace the winter months with a renewed spirit and balanced perspective. As you fold yoga into your daily routine, you may find it not just a seasonal remedy but a lifelong companion in the journey toward holistic health.

7.2 THE ROLE OF ACUPUNCTURE IN TREATING SEASONAL AFFECTIVE DISORDER

In the realm of alternative medicine, acupuncture stands out as a venerable practice with roots deeply embedded in the traditions of Traditional Chinese Medicine (TCM). This ancient practice is based on the concept of Qi (pronounced "chi"), which is understood as the vital life force or energy that flows through the body. According to TCM, the disruption or imbalance of Qi can lead to various health issues, including emotional disorders like Seasonal Affective Disorder (SAD). Acupuncture seeks to restore balance to this flow of energy by inserting fine, sterile needles into specific points along the body's energy pathways, known as meridians. The stimulation of these points is believed to enhance the body's natural healing capabilities and restore equilibrium to the physical and emotional aspects of the individual. For those grappling with SAD, acupuncture offers a promising avenue for alleviating the symptoms and for addressing the energetic imbalances that may underlie the condition, promoting a deeper sense of well-being and balance throughout the challenging winter months.

The efficacy of acupuncture in treating SAD is increasingly supported by contemporary research that bridges Eastern practices with Western scientific methodologies. Studies have indicated that acupuncture can influence the regulation of neurotransmitters such as serotonin and melatonin, which play significant roles in mood regulation and sleep patterns—both of which are essential elements affected in SAD. Patient experiences often reflect a reduction in common symptoms of SAD, such as persistent low mood, fatigue, and sleep disturbances, following regular acupuncture treatments. Clinical outcomes also suggest improvements in emotional well-being, with many reporting enhanced feelings of relaxation and vitality. These findings are compelling, not only for their immediate implications for symptom relief but also for their potential to offer a long-term strategy for managing SAD without the reliance on pharmacological interventions, which may carry side effects or interact with other medications.

Understanding what to expect during an acupuncture treatment can help demystify the process, making it more accessible for those considering this therapy. Typically, an initial session with a licensed acupuncturist will involve a comprehensive assessment of your health history and current symptoms, followed by the formulation of a treatment plan tailored to your specific needs. During the treatment, needles are gently inserted into selected acupoints, which might be far from the parts of the body where symptoms are manifesting, as acupuncture views the body holistically. The needles are usually retained for about 20 to 30 minutes while you lie still and possibly experience a state of deep relaxation or even sleep. Treatment frequency can vary, but many practitioners recommend starting with weekly sessions, gradually extending the interval between sessions as symptoms improve.

Integrating acupuncture into a broader treatment plan for SAD involves a holistic approach that includes lifestyle adjustments, dietary changes, and possibly other therapeutic modalities. For example, combining acupuncture with light therapy may enhance the overall effectiveness, with acupuncture strengthening the body's internal balance and light therapy addressing the lack of sunlight exposure directly linked to SAD. Dietary recommendations based on TCM principles, such as incorporating warming and nourishing foods during the colder months, can also support the body's Yin-Yang balance, contributing to emotional and physical wellness. Engaging in regular physical activity, maintaining a healthy sleep schedule, and participating in social activities can complement the benefits of acupuncture, creating a comprehensive and personalized strategy for managing SAD effectively. By considering all aspects of health—physical, emotional, and environmental—this integrative approach targets the symptoms of SAD, enhancing overall resilience and quality of life, making it a robust framework for those seeking to overcome the seasonal challenges posed by this condition.

7.3 ART AND MUSIC THERAPY: CREATIVE OUTLETS FOR MANAGING SYMPTOMS

In the quiet corners of a world often dominated by clinical treatments and medication, art and music therapy emerge as vibrant beacons of hope for those grappling with Seasonal Affective Disorder (SAD). These forms of expressive therapy serve not merely as distractions but as profound channels for emotional expression and processing. The act of creating art or engaging in musical activities can be incredibly therapeutic, providing a nonverbal outlet for emotions that are often complex and difficult to articulate. This process of creation can lead to significant emotional release, helping to alleviate some of the heavy burdens that SAD imposes.

Art therapy involves the use of creative techniques in a huge variety of media, such as drawing, painting, collage, coloring, and sculpting, to name a few. As individuals express themselves artistically, they can examine the psychological and emotional undertones in their art. For someone dealing with SAD, this can mean an opportunity to externalize feelings of sadness, anxiety, or lethargy that are challenging to express in words, thus making them more manageable. Music therapy, similarly, uses music to address physical, emotional, cognitive, and social needs, incorporating elements like listening to melodies, playing an instrument, drumming, or writing songs. The rhythmic and melodic aspects of music are known to facilitate relaxation, improve mood, and decrease anxiety, all of which are beneficial in managing the symptoms of SAD.

Case Studies and Applications

Several case studies highlight the effectiveness of art and music therapy in managing SAD. In one instance, a group of individuals diagnosed with SAD participated in weekly art therapy sessions over the winter months. Many reported significant reductions in their depressive symptoms, noting that creating art provided them with a sense of accomplishment and temporary relief from their usual state of lethargy and sadness. Another case involved the use of music therapy where patients engaged in group singing sessions. Participants noted improvements in mood and social connectivity, which are often negatively impacted by SAD. These examples underscore the potential of art and music therapy not only as tools for emotional expression but also for fostering a sense of community and shared experience among those affected by SAD.

Accessing Therapeutic Resources

Finding qualified art and music therapists can be an integral step in integrating these therapies into a treatment plan for SAD. Certified therapists are trained to guide individuals through the creative process in a way that maximizes therapeutic benefits. You can locate licensed practitioners through professional associations such as the American Art Therapy Association and the American Music Therapy Association. These organizations provide directories of professionals by area, ensuring you can find a therapist whose expertise aligns with your needs. There are many community centers, hospitals, and clinics that recognize the value of these therapies and offer programs specifically designed for individuals dealing with mental health issues, including SAD.

DIY Approaches for Home

For those who may not have immediate access to professional art or music therapists, there are several do-it-yourself approaches that can be beneficial. Setting aside a personal space at home for engaging in art or music can be a great start. This could involve creating a small art studio corner with supplies for drawing, painting, or crafting, or an area with musical instruments that are easily accessible. Engaging regularly in these activities can help structure your day and provide meaningful distraction from the cyclical thoughts often associated with SAD. Additionally, online tutorials and apps offer guided sessions in both art and music therapy, allowing you to explore these therapeutic avenues from the comfort of your own home.

Art and music therapy provide powerful avenues for managing the symptoms of Seasonal Affective Disorder, offering both creative expression and emotional relief. These therapies underscore the importance of holistic approaches in the treatment of SAD, reminding us that healing can often be found in the harmony of a melody or the stroke of a paintbrush. As you explore these expressive therapies, whether through professional guidance or personal exploration, you may discover a reduction in your symptoms and a profound connection to a form of expression that resonates with your journey through the seasons.

7.4 HERBAL REMEDIES AND THEIR PLACE IN SAD MANAGEMENT

In the quiet, often introspective battle against Seasonal Affective Disorder (SAD), many find solace and relief in the natural world, particularly through herbal remedies known for their mood-supportive properties. The use of herbs like St. John's Wort and SAM-e has been rooted in traditional practices for centuries, and their modern applications continue to be supported by growing scientific research. These herbal supplements are not just remnants of ancient medicine; rather, they are components of a contemporary holistic approach to managing mood disorders, offering a natural complement to light therapy and pharmacological treatments.

St. John's Wort, scientifically known as Hypericum perforatum, is one of the most well-known herbs for combating depressive symptoms, and its effectiveness extends to those specifically associated with SAD. Renowned for its ability to enhance mood, St. John's Wort operates by influencing neurotransmitters involved in mood regulation, such as serotonin, dopamine, and norepinephrine. This herb is particularly favored for its dual impact on mood and sleep, addressing two of the major challenges faced by individuals dealing with SAD. Meanwhile, SAM-e (S-adenosylmethionine), a compound naturally produced by the body that can also be taken in supplement form, has been noted for its swift impact on alleviating depressive symptoms. It is involved in the synthesis of neurotransmitters, and its additional role in supporting joint health and liver function makes it a multifaceted supplement, beneficial in the holistic management of SAD.

While the potential benefits of these herbal remedies are compelling, integrating them into your SAD management plan requires careful consideration. The interaction of these supplements with other treatments, particularly prescription medications for depression or anxiety, can pose risks. For instance, St. John's Wort is known to interact with a variety of pharmaceuticals, potentially diminishing their effectiveness or leading to unwanted side effects. Therefore, the integration of herbal treatments should always be approached with a strategy that emphasizes safety and efficacy. This involves not only being aware of potential interactions but also understanding the appropriate dosages and durations for use. Working closely with a healthcare provider who understands both herbal and conventional medical treatments is highly recommended. With an informed and balanced perspective, working with your healthcare provider, you can determine if and when to incorporate these remedies into your overall treatment plan.

The growing body of scientific evidence supporting the use of herbal remedies for SAD adds an important layer of credibility to their use. Numerous studies have explored the efficacy of St. John's Wort in treating mild to moderate depression, with many findings suggesting it may be as effective as some standard antidepressants for these conditions. Similarly, research into SAM-e has indicated its potential for quick improvement in depressive symptoms, often showing results within just a few days. However, it's vital to critically evaluate this research, recognizing the variability in study designs and the differences in individual responses to herbal treatment. This scrutiny ensures that you are making informed decisions based on reliable information, tailored to your specific circumstances and health profile.

Given the complexities and potential risks associated with herbal remedies, the importance of consulting with healthcare professionals cannot be overstated. This consultation should go beyond merely obtaining approval to use these supplements; it should be an opportunity to discuss your overall health, other treatments you're undergoing, and the specific symptoms you're aiming to manage. A healthcare provider who is knowledgeable in both conventional and alternative medicine can provide guidance on the optimal use of herbal supplements, helping you to navigate potential interactions and adjust dosages as needed to safely and effectively incorporate these natural remedies into your SAD management strategy. This professional guidance ensures that your approach to managing SAD is comprehensive and specifically tailored to support your health and well-being across all aspects of life.

7.5 THE IMPACT OF SOCIAL ACTIVITIES AND VOLUNTEERING ON SAD

The winter season, with its shorter days and colder weather, can often lead to feelings of isolation and melancholy, particularly for those experiencing Seasonal Affective Disorder (SAD). Engaging in social activities and volunteering can serve as a therapeutic antidote, providing a distraction from the dreariness of the season, as well as offering profound benefits in terms of emotional and psychological health. The act of connecting with others through meaningful activities can foster a sense of purpose and community, vital components often diminished by the symptoms of SAD. When you volunteer or participate in group activities, you step outside the solitary confines of your daily routine, which can be especially monotonous and lonely during the winter months. This engagement provides needed social interaction, which stimulates the production of neurotransmitters like endorphins and serotonin, enhancing mood and overall feelings of well-being.

Finding activities that resonate with your interests and provide a sense of achievement can transform the winter months from a time of endurance to one of enjoyment and personal growth. Start by identifying local community centers, non-profits, or clubs that align with your passions or hobbies. Whether it's a book club, a cooking class, or a local theater group, these organized settings provide structured opportunities to interact with others who share similar interests, making the social interactions easier and more rewarding. Additionally, many communities offer seasonal events like winter markets or festivals, which can be excellent opportunities to engage with your local community in a festive, relaxed environment. Engaging in these activities fills your social calendar and gives you events to look forward to. They also help you build a supportive network of acquaintances who can turn into friends, reinforcing your social support system.

Volunteering, in particular, can be incredibly beneficial during the winter months, as it provides structured social interaction and a positive focus that can counteract the feelings of uselessness or guilt that often accompany SAD. By focusing on helping others, you shift your perspective outward, which can alleviate self-focused rumination and depressive thoughts. Look for opportunities that match your skills and interests to ensure the experience is mutually beneficial. For instance, if you enjoy animals, volunteering at a local animal shelter could provide the dual benefits of social interaction and the uplifting presence of animals, which have been shown to improve mood and reduce stress. Similarly, volunteering at a food bank or a community kitchen involves working with a team and provides the intrinsic reward of knowing you're contributing to the well-being of those less fortunate, enhancing your sense of purpose and self-worth.

Balancing these activities with the need for self-care and downtime is needed, especially for individuals managing SAD. It's important to listen to your body and recognize when you might be overextending yourself. Engaging too heavily in social activities can lead to burnout, particularly if your energy levels are already compromised by the shorter daylight hours. Establish a balanced schedule that allows for regular social interaction without compromising your need for quiet, restorative time. This might mean prioritizing certain activities that provide the most benefit and learning to say no to others that may be too demanding. Additionally, integrating relaxation practices such as meditation or gentle yoga on days when you're not actively volunteering or participating in social events can help maintain a healthy balance between activity and rest.

In embracing social activities and volunteering as part of your strategy to manage SAD, you enrich your winter experience, transforming it from a season to endure into a season to enjoy and anticipate. The connections made, and the satisfaction gained from these engagements can provide immediate relief from the symptoms of SAD, build resilience and a supportive community that extends beyond the winter months, enhancing your overall quality of life.

7.6 EXPLORING LIGHT AND COLOR THERAPY BEYOND TRADITIONAL LIGHT BOXES

The landscape of light therapy, a cornerstone in treating Seasonal Affective Disorder (SAD), is evolving rapidly, transcending beyond the confines of traditional light boxes to embrace more dynamic and versatile forms. Innovations in this field are not just enhancing the efficacy of light therapy but are also making it more accessible and integrated into everyday lives. Among these advancements, wearable light therapy devices stand out for their convenience and adaptability. These devices, which can range from visors to glasses, emit a light spectrum similar to daylight and are designed to be used on the go. This mobility allows for a more natural integration of light therapy into daily routines, making it less intrusive and more consistent with modern lifestyles. Similarly, ambient lighting solutions, which adjust the light in an environment to mimic natural outdoor conditions, are gaining traction. These systems can be programmed to change intensity and color temperature throughout the day, aligning indoor lighting with the body's circadian rhythm, thus supporting better mood and sleep patterns.

Color Therapy Basics

Delving into the realm of color therapy offers another layer of nuance in managing mood disorders like SAD. Rooted in the principle that different colors can evoke different psychological, emotional, and physical responses, color therapy—or chromotherapy—utilizes these effects to improve mental health and mood. For instance, blue light is often used in light therapy for its ability to regulate circadian rhythms and improve alertness, making it beneficial for those experiencing SAD. On the other hand, warmer colors like red and orange are believed to boost energy and vitality, which can be particularly helpful during the low-energy months of winter. Integrating color therapy into daily life can be as simple as changing the bulbs in your home to emit different colors, or using devices like color therapy lamps that allow for customized settings depending on your mood and the time of day.

Customizing Light Environments

Creating a personalized light environment in your home or workspace can significantly enhance your ability to manage SAD. Start by assessing the natural light availability in your living or working areas. Maximizing natural light exposure by arranging seating areas near windows or using light-reflective decor can help alleviate symptoms of SAD. For darker spaces or days when natural light is insufficient, consider installing adjustable light therapy lamps that allow you to modify intensity and color temperature according to your specific needs. There are several companies and styles of light fixtures on Amazon that have higher than 4-star reviews with a whole range of price points. Companies such as Luminette, Lastar, Aoife Light Therapy, Verilux, Circadian Optics, Alaska Northern Lights, and Day Light Therapy to name a few. Smart home systems that automate lighting based on time of day can also be an excellent investment, ensuring that you receive optimal light exposure without having to constantly adjust settings manually. These customized environments may cater to your therapeutic needs and enhance overall well-being by creating spaces that feel comfortable and uplifting.

Combining Light and Color Therapies

The synergistic potential of combining light and color therapies opens up a comprehensive approach to managing SAD. This integration involves using both the intensity and color properties of light to simulate natural daylight variations, providing holistic benefits. For example, using a light fixture that emits full-spectrum light in the morning can help reset your circadian rhythm, while limiting colors like green or blue in the evening can aid in relaxation and readiness for sleep. This dual strategy addresses the biological underpinnings of SAD by regulating melatonin and serotonin levels and also enhances the psychological aspects of color perception, which can influence mood and emotional well-being. To implement this combined approach effectively, consider consulting a therapist who specializes in environmental therapies. They can provide guidance on the optimal light and color combinations and help tailor a regimen that fits seamlessly into your daily routine, maximizing therapeutic outcomes.

As we wrap up this exploration of innovative light and color therapies for SAD, it's clear that the options for creating healing environments are more diverse and accessible than ever. These therapies, whether used individually or in combination, offer powerful tools for enhancing mood, energy, and overall well-being during the challenging winter months. As we continue to uncover and integrate these therapeutic innovations, the potential for managing SAD more effectively and holistically grows, promising a brighter outlook for those affected by seasonal mood variations. Looking ahead, the next chapter will delve into personal stories of resilience and recovery, providing real-life insights and inspiration for navigating life with Seasonal Affective Disorder.

8

EMPOWERMENT AND HOPE

As the first snowflakes of winter whisper against the windowpane, a reminder of the season's beauty and its challenges, many face the onset of Seasonal Affective Disorder (SAD) with a sense of trepidation. Yet, amidst the frost and the shorter days, there lies an opportunity—a chance to forge a path of personal empowerment and proactive management of SAD. This chapter is dedicated to transforming how you interact with this pervasive disorder, guiding you through creating a personalized management plan that resonates with your unique life circumstances and needs.

8.1 DEVELOPING A PERSONALIZED SAD MANAGEMENT PLAN

Individual Needs Assessment

Embarking on the journey to manage SAD effectively begins with a thorough assessment of your individual needs and symptoms.

This process is akin to mapping the terrain of your personal experience with SAD—identifying the specific symptoms that challenge you most, the times of day when you feel most vulnerable, and the activities that either exacerbate or alleviate your condition. This detailed understanding forms the foundation of your personalized management plan. It's important to consider factors such as your daily responsibilities, your physical environment, and your previous experiences with SAD treatments. By aligning this plan with your personal history and current lifestyle, you ensure the strategies you adopt are effective and sustainable.

Incorporating Various Treatments

With your unique profile in hand, the next step is to weave together various treatments into a cohesive management plan. Light therapy, a cornerstone in treating SAD, might be your starting point, utilizing specially designed lamps to mimic natural sunlight and help reset your biological clock. However, the complexity of SAD often requires a multi-faceted approach. Medications such as SSRIs can be discussed with your healthcare provider to manage severe symptoms, while psychotherapy, particularly Cognitive Behavioral Therapy (CBT), is effective in addressing the cognitive aspects of SAD. Lifestyle adjustments play a crucial role as well; regular exercise, a nutritious diet, and sufficient sleep are all vital components. Integrating these treatments requires careful coordination—considering how each component fits into your daily routine and interacts with others. For instance, timing light therapy sessions to complement your sleep schedule and medication timings can enhance overall effectiveness.

Setting Realistic Goals

Within your management plan, setting realistic, achievable goals is the basis for sustainability. These goals act as beacons—guiding your path and providing motivation. Start with small, manageable objectives, such as incorporating a 30-minute walk into your morning routine or using the light therapy lamp every day for two weeks. Celebrate these small victories, as they build your confidence and reinforce your commitment to managing SAD. As you become more comfortable and adept at managing your daily strategies, you can expand your goals to include longer-term aspirations, such as strengthening your relationships or pursuing new hobbies which were previously hindered by SAD.

Review and Adaptation

Finally, the dynamic nature of life and SAD itself means that your management plan must be adaptable. Regular review sessions, perhaps at the change of seasons or at scheduled intervals with your therapist, provide opportunities to reflect on what's working and what isn't. This adaptability ensures that your management plan remains aligned with your evolving needs and continues to provide the best support possible. Changes in lifestyle, unexpected stressors, or shifts in your symptoms might all necessitate adjustments to your plan. Embracing this flexibility allows you to maintain control over your management of SAD, empowering you to make proactive changes that support your well-being.

Through these detailed steps—assessment, integration, goal setting, and adaptation—you create a living document, although keeping a written journal to track your progress maybe beneficial as well. Your personalized SAD management plan serves to manage the condition and enhance your life despite it. This plan is not static; it evolves as you do, a testament to your resilience and proactive stance against Seasonal Affective Disorder. As you move forward, each step you take is a step towards a brighter, more balanced life, even amidst the challenges of SAD.

8.2 SUCCESS STORIES: OVERCOMING SAD AND THRIVING

Amidst the frigid embrace of winter, when the sun's warmth seems but a distant memory, the stories of those who have faced and overcome Seasonal Affective Disorder (SAD) shine as beacons of hope and resilience. These narratives offer inspiration and serve as valuable roadmaps for others navigating the icy clutches of this condition. Let's delve into the experiences of individuals who have turned their struggle with SAD into a journey of self-discovery and empowerment, each story unfolding unique paths to wellness that resonate with universal themes of perseverance and transformation.

Consider the tale of Maria, a graphic designer whose life seemed to pause every winter as SAD clouded her days with unshakeable lethargy and melancholy. Determined to reclaim her vibrancy, Maria embarked on a multifaceted treatment approach that included light therapy, guided meditation, and a structured exercise regimen. The turning point came when she joined a local support group for individuals with SAD, where she found not only solace but also a sense of purpose. Sharing her own experiences and coping strategies became Maria's gateway to empowerment. Her story underscores a valuable lesson: holistic treatment supported by a compassionate community can catalyze profound personal growth and recovery. Maria's journey reveals the transformative power of community support, highlighting how shared experiences can amplify individual healing processes.

Then there's the story of James, a retired school teacher whose encounter with SAD later in life took him by surprise. James felt confined by the walls of his home as the shorter days rolled in, his zest for life dimming as swiftly as the daylight. His breakthrough came through a combination of vitamin D supplementation and cognitive behavioral therapy, which helped him reframe his negative thoughts about the winter months. However, it was his decision to volunteer at a local shelter that infused his winter days with renewed meaning and connection. James's experience illustrates another vital lesson: engaging in altruistic activities can significantly mitigate the symptoms of SAD by fostering connections and enhancing one's sense of worth and community contribution.

Each story of overcoming SAD is also a testament to the indispensable role of support networks, encompassing both formal mental health support and informal social connections. These networks provide emotional sustenance, practical advice, and shared experiences that can ease the sense of isolation that often accompanies SAD. The encouragement and understanding from a support group can fortify one's resolve to adhere to treatment plans, while friends and family offer daily strength and motivation. This collective support is vital, acting as both a cushion and a catalyst in the journey toward wellness.

Drawing from these narratives, we distill essential insights that can guide others in their own paths to managing SAD. From Maria's and James's stories, we learn the importance of a proactive approach—adopting therapeutic practices and seeking out community connections before the winter season fully sets in. We also see the value of flexibility, as both found that adjusting their strategies over time was necessary to match their evolving needs and responses to treatments. Their experiences highlight that while SAD is a formidable foe, it can also be a powerful teacher—

prompting individuals to explore new hobbies, forge new relationships, and ultimately, discover new strengths.

These stories illuminate paths to managing SAD and transform the narrative around living with a seasonal disorder. They shift the focus from enduring to thriving, demonstrating how each challenge overcome adds a layer of resilience and self-awareness. For anyone grappling with SAD, these stories are a reminder that you are not alone in your struggle, and that with the right tools and support, you can navigate even the toughest winters—and emerge stronger and more connected to those around you.

8.3 STAYING INFORMED: KEEPING UP WITH SAD RESEARCH AND DEVELOPMENTS

In a field as dynamic as mental health, staying informed about the latest research and developments in Seasonal Affective Disorder (SAD) is not just beneficial—it's necessary for anyone looking to manage their condition effectively. With new studies and findings frequently emerging, understanding the current trends in SAD research can significantly enhance your ability to make informed decisions about your health. Researchers continue to explore various aspects of SAD, ranging from its biological bases to the effectiveness of new treatment modalities. For instance, recent studies have begun to shed light on the genetic factors that may predispose individuals to SAD, offering a more in-depth understanding of the disorder and potential avenues for personalized treatment strategies.

To navigate this wealth of information, identifying reliable sources is foundational. Medical journals such as the "Journal of Affective Disorders" and "Psychiatry Research" regularly publish peer-reviewed articles on the latest SAD research. These journals provide insights from studies conducted by leading experts in the field, ensuring that the information is both accurate and up-to-date. Additionally, organizations like the National Institute of Mental Health (NIMH) offer resources and updates on their websites, making it easier for non-specialists to access and understand important findings. Trusted websites such as Mayo Clinic and WebMD also provide summaries of recent research, often with commentary from medical professionals to help contextualize the information.

Applying this research to your daily life and management plan requires a discerning approach. It's important to not only read about new findings but also to evaluate their relevance and applicability to your situation. For example, if a new study suggests that a particular type of light therapy is especially effective, consider how this might fit into your existing treatment regimen. Could this be an opportunity to experiment with a new device or technique? Consulting with your healthcare provider can help interpret these findings and decide whether they warrant a change in your treatment strategy. This collaborative approach ensures that any modifications to your management plan are made thoughtfully, based on solid research and tailored to your specific needs.

Moreover, engaging with the SAD community and healthcare professionals can enrich your understanding and application of new research. Many cities and online platforms host forums, workshops, and conferences that focus on SAD and general mental health. These venues provide opportunities to connect with others who share similar experiences, exchange ideas, and discuss the latest research and treatment options. Such interactions can also inspire community-led initiatives or support groups, fostering a proactive approach to managing SAD. Healthcare professionals, particularly those specializing in mood disorders, are invaluable resources for discussing new research and therapeutic strategies. They can provide insights into how emerging trends might benefit your particular case, offering a professional perspective that complements your personal research.

Navigating the evolving landscape of SAD research empowers you to make informed decisions about your health and treatment options. By staying updated, critically assessing information, and engaging with both professionals and the community, you ensure that your approach to managing SAD is as effective and informed as possible. This proactive stance enhances your ability to cope with the disorder and contributes to a more profound understanding of SAD, driving a more informed and supportive community response to this challenging condition. As you continue to adapt and refine your management strategies, let the latest research illuminate your path, offering hope and guidance as you navigate the complexities of Seasonal Affective Disorder.

8.4 ADVOCATING FOR SAD AWARENESS IN YOUR COMMUNITY

Raising awareness about Seasonal Affective Disorder (SAD) within your community is essential for fostering a supportive environment as well as ensuring that those affected receive the understanding and help they need. Initiating and participating in public awareness campaigns can dramatically change the landscape of how SAD is perceived and treated. Organizing community talks is a powerful way to start these conversations. These talks can be set up in local libraries, schools, or community centers, where experts like psychologists or experienced therapists present key information about SAD. They can share insights on symptoms, treatments, and effective management strategies, helping to demystify the disorder and reduce associated stigma. Incorporating interactive elements such as question-and-answer sessions can engage the audience more directly, allowing for a deeper understanding and personal connection to the information presented.

Social media campaigns can also play a vital role in raising awareness. Platforms like Facebook, Instagram, and X (formerly known as Twitter), offer extensive reach and the ability to connect with a broad audience quickly. Creating informative posts, sharing personal stories, and linking to reliable sources of information about SAD can help spread awareness efficiently. These posts can be scheduled to coincide with the onset of shorter days in early autumn when SAD symptoms typically begin to appear, maximizing their relevance and impact. Engaging infographics that outline symptoms or simple steps for managing SAD can be particularly effective, as they are easily shareable and can visually communicate important information at a glance.

Educational workshops complement these efforts by providing detailed, actionable information in an interactive format. These workshops can cover topics such as coping strategies, nutritional advice to combat SAD, or demonstrations of light therapy usage. Inviting mental health professionals to lead these workshops ensures that the information is accurate and beneficial. Moreover, workshops can be tailored to specific groups within the community, such as parents, educators, or healthcare professionals, to address the unique ways in which SAD impacts different segments of the population.

Engaging healthcare providers in your community is another important aspect of advocating for better SAD support and understanding. This engagement can be facilitated through informational sessions specifically designed for healthcare professionals, where the latest research and treatment options are discussed. Encouraging local practitioners to incorporate screening for SAD into routine examinations can lead to earlier diagnosis and treatment, significantly improving outcomes for patients. Building relationships with these providers ensures that they have the resources and knowledge necessary to support individuals struggling with SAD effectively.

Supporting policy change is necessary for creating a community that accommodates the needs of those with SAD. This could involve advocating for more flexible work or school hours to accommodate light therapy schedules, or pushing for insurance plans to cover treatments such as counseling and light therapy devices. Engaging with local government representatives to discuss these changes can lead to broader community support and legislative action. Preparing clear, concise presentations that outline the benefits of such policies not only for individuals with SAD but for community well-being overall can facilitate more significant consideration and action from policymakers.

Finally, building a community network or group focused on SAD awareness and advocacy can provide a sustained, collective voice for these efforts. This network can coordinate the various activities mentioned, from awareness campaigns to policy advocacy, ensuring that efforts are continuous and consistent. Regular meetings can help plan activities, share resources, and offer support to members affected by SAD. Such a network strengthens the community's capacity to support its members and can serve as a model for similar initiatives in other communities.

Through these multifaceted efforts—public education, social media engagement, targeted workshops, healthcare provider involvement, policy advocacy, and community networking—you can significantly enhance awareness and understanding of SAD in your community. These initiatives educate the public and build a supportive framework that can profoundly impact those affected by Seasonal Affective Disorder, fostering a community environment where compassion and understanding pave the way for effective management and support.

8.5 THE FUTURE OF SAD TREATMENT: WHAT'S ON THE HORIZON?

As we look toward the future of managing Seasonal Affective Disorder (SAD), a wave of innovation and more in-depth understanding promises to reshape our approach to this pervasive condition. The horizon is bright with emerging treatments and technologies that enhance the efficacy of traditional methods, and open new avenues for personalized and holistic care. One of the most exciting developments is the advent of advanced light therapy devices. These are not your standard light boxes; they are smarter, more user-friendly, and integrated with technology that adjusts light exposure based on individual response patterns. Imagine devices that learn from your daily mood fluctuations and adjust their output to provide optimal support for your specific circadian rhythm. This level of personalization extends beyond convenience, offering the potential to significantly boost the effectiveness of light therapy with precision that was previously unattainable.

The realm of genetic research in SAD treatment is also expanding, providing fascinating insights that could lead to highly personalized treatment plans. Scientists are delving into the genetic markers that may predispose individuals to SAD, exploring how these markers influence the body's response to changes in light and season. This research is paving the way for treatments that are tailored not just to the symptoms but to the genetic profile of the individual. Imagine a scenario where a simple genetic test could guide your doctor in customizing a treatment plan that is the most effective for your specific genetic makeup, potentially enhancing the response to treatment and minimizing side effects.

The integration of holistic and integrative approaches is set to play a larger role in the treatment of SAD. This holistic view encompasses not only the physical symptoms but also the psychological and social aspects of health. Treatments that include mindfulness practices, dietary adjustments, and even the architectural design of living spaces to maximize natural light are becoming more mainstream. These methods acknowledge the complex interplay of factors that influence mental health and emphasize the importance of a supportive environment as part of the treatment plan. The future of SAD treatment looks to these integrative strategies to provide a more comprehensive approach that aligns with general well-being and preventive health care.

Furthermore, global perspectives on SAD are enriching our understanding and approaches to treatment. International collaborations in research are uncovering how SAD affects populations in different geographical locations, leading to an in-depth understanding of the global impact of this disorder. These collaborations are paramount as they integrate diverse perspectives and expertise, leading to more innovative and effective solutions that can be adapted to various cultural contexts. For example, the way SAD is treated in Nordic countries, where the disorder is widely recognized and research is robust, can offer insights and strategies that might be applied in places where SAD is less known or underresearched.

These advancements in treatment technologies, genetic research, holistic approaches, and global collaboration are transforming the landscape of SAD management. As we continue to embrace and integrate these innovations, the future holds promising potential for individuals affected by Seasonal Affective Disorder to find more effective, personalized, and comprehensive support. This forward-thinking approach aims to mitigate the symptoms associated with SAD and enhances overall life quality. This will pave the way for a future where the cold and dark months can be faced not with dread, but with a well-equipped, resilient outlook.

8.6 EMBRACING YOUR JOURNEY WITH SAD: A MESSAGE OF HOPE

In the quiet solitude that often accompanies the colder months, it's easy to view Seasonal Affective Disorder (SAD) solely as a formidable foe. Yet, within this challenge lies a profound opportunity for personal evolution and discovery. Embracing your experience with SAD isn't about merely coping with symptoms; it's about recognizing this part of your life as a catalyst for growth and self-awareness. Each winter can serve as a chapter in your ongoing story of resilience, where you learn more about your needs, boundaries, and strengths.

Acceptance is huge in this process. It involves acknowledging SAD as a significant influence in your life but not the defining one. By accepting the disorder, you open yourself up to the full range of experiences and emotions it brings, without judgment. This acceptance is the first step towards using your experience as a tool for growth. It allows you to observe how your feelings and behaviors change with the seasons, giving you valuable insights into your personal patterns and triggers. This knowledge is powerful. It equips you to make more informed decisions about your care and to adjust your lifestyle in ways that honor your needs.

Vulnerability, often seen as a weakness, is actually a reservoir of strength, especially for those managing SAD. Sharing your story isn't just about unburdening yourself or seeking support; it's an act of courage that can profoundly impact others. Your experiences can light the way for someone else in the darkness of their struggle, showing them they are not alone. This sharing creates a network of understanding and support, a community where people are bound not just by shared challenges, but by shared strength and resilience. Each story shared adds another layer of collective knowledge and empathy, enriching the community's ability to support each other.

Living with SAD is indeed a continuous journey, marked by ebbs and flows, triumphs, and setbacks. It's impactful to celebrate each step forward, no matter how small. These celebrations act as affirmations of your resilience; they reinforce your ability to manage the disorder and thrive despite it. Whether it's a particularly productive day, or a week when you managed to exercise regularly, or simply a moment when you felt genuine joy during the winter months—each is a victory worth recognizing. These moments build on one another, creating a momentum that can carry you through tougher times.

Hope and resilience are perhaps the most vital aspects of managing SAD. They remind you that with the right strategies and supports, not only is it possible to live well with SAD, but it's also possible to lead a vibrant, fulfilling life. This disorder, while certainly challenging, does not have the power to define your existence. It is one part of a complex, beautiful life filled with potential. With each year, as you learn more and refine your management strategies, you build resilience—not just against SAD but against any of life's challenges. This resilience is a testament to your strength and adaptability, qualities that shine brightly even during the shortest days of winter.

As this chapter closes, remember that your journey with SAD is uniquely yours. It is a path paved with challenges, but also with profound opportunities for growth and connection. Each step you take builds knowledge, strength, and resilience, contributing to a fuller understanding of yourself and the disorder. This journey is not just about managing symptoms but about transforming them into avenues for personal discovery and empowerment. As you continue to navigate your path, let hope light your way, and may resilience be your steadfast companion. Now, as we turn to the conclusion of this book, let's reflect on the key insights and strategies that can help you and your loved ones not just endure but thrive, no matter the season.

CONCLUSION

As we draw the curtains on this enlightening journey through the pages of this book, let us take a moment to reflect on the path we have traveled together. Starting with the basics of Seasonal Affective Disorder, we ventured into the complexities of its symptoms, diagnosis, and the pervasive myths that cloud its understanding. Your engagement and curiosity have allowed us to explore a myriad of treatment and management strategies, delve into the importance of support systems, and embrace holistic approaches that go beyond conventional medical treatments.

Understanding SAD has been at the core of our discussion, recognizing it as a significant mental health condition that touches many lives, often hidden behind the veil of seasonal changes. We've uncovered how SAD is more than just "winter blues" and demands serious attention and tailored management strategies.

Empowerment through knowledge has been a recurring theme, highlighting how necessary it is for those affected by SAD, and their loved ones, to advocate for themselves with confidence. Armed with the insights from this book, you are now better equipped to make informed decisions that enhance your well-being or that of someone you care about.

However, it's imperative to remember that **managing SAD is a deeply personal journey**. I encourage you to adapt the strategies discussed to align with your unique circumstances. The effectiveness of treatments varies from person to person; thus, personalizing your approach is key to finding what works best for you.

As you continue on your path, I urge you to **remain proactive in educating yourself about SAD**. Stay updated with the latest research and emerging treatments. The landscape of mental health is ever-evolving, and staying informed is your best defense. Moreover, become an advocate for SAD awareness in your community. Share your knowledge and experiences to help destigmatize mental health issues and foster a supportive environment where everyone can seek the help they need without fear of judgment.

Finally, let me offer you **words of hope and encouragement**: managing SAD effectively is entirely possible. With the right tools, information, and community support, you can navigate through the darker months with resilience and joy. Remember, each small step you take in understanding and managing this disorder illuminates a path not just for you, but also for others who might be silently struggling.

I want to express my heartfelt **thanks to you, the reader** for embarking on this journey with me. Your willingness to dive deep into the world of Seasonal Affective Disorder, to learn, understand, and perhaps apply this newfound knowledge, is a powerful step toward a brighter, more balanced life. Please share this knowledge with others who might be walking through life unaware of the name of the shadow they fight every winter.

Together, let's spread light and hope. I would greatly appreciate it if you would leave a review.

May this book serve as a beacon during your moments of doubt and a reminder that even amidst the challenges of SAD, a fulfilling life awaits. With each page you turned, you gathered more strength, and with every chapter, you armed yourself with knowledge. Carry these with you as tools of empowerment and symbols of your commitment to thriving, no matter the season.

REFERENCES

- *Seasonal Affective Disorder* https://www.nimh.nih.gov/health/publications/seasonal-affective-disorder
- *Effect of Light on Human Circadian Physiology - PMC* https://www.ncbi.nlm.nih.gov/pmc/articles/PMC2717723/
- *Seasonal Affective Disorder (SAD): More Than the Winter Blues* https://www.nimh.nih.gov/health/publications/seasonal-affective-disorder-sad-more-than-the-winter-blues
- *An epidemiological study on gender differences in self ...* https://pubmed.ncbi.nlm.nih.gov/16195086/#:~
- *Bright Light Therapy: Seasonal Affective Disorder and ...* https://www.ncbi.nlm.nih.gov/pmc/articles/PMC6746555/
- *Treatment of seasonal affective disorders - PMC* https://www.ncbi.nlm.nih.gov/pmc/articles/PMC3181778/
- *CBT for Seasonal Affective Disorder* https://www.mindbody7.com/news/2017/12/7/cognitive-behavioral-therapy-for-seasonal-affective-disorder
- *Omega-3 fatty acids for mood disorders* https://www.health.harvard.edu/blog/omega-3-fatty-acids-for-mood-disorders-2018080314414
- *Why Natural Light Is Important for Mental and Physical Health* https://delos.com/blog/why-natural-light-is-important-for-mental-and-physical-health/
- *What to Know About Meditation and Depression - WebMD* https://www.webmd.com/depression/what-to-know-about-meditation-and-depression
- *9 Workouts to Help Lift Winter Blues* https://www.tonal.com/blog/9-workouts-to-help-lift-winter-blues/
- *Nutritional & lifestyle changes to support SAD* https://foodforthebrain.org/sad-how-to-prevent-and-manage-symptoms-with-nutrition-and-lifestyle-changes/
- *Seasonal affective disorder (SAD)* https://www.mind.org.uk/information-support/types-of-mental-health-problems/seasonal-affective-disorder-sad/for-friends-and-family/

- *Communication strategies to counter stigma and improve ...* https://www.ncbi.nlm.nih.gov/pmc/articles/PMC5794622/
- *Seasonal affective disorder (SAD) - Diagnosis & treatment* https://www.mayoclinic.org/diseases-conditions/seasonal-affective-disorder/diagnosis-treatment/drc-20364722
- *Self-Care for Caregivers of Mental Health Patients* https://www.aic.sg/caregiving/self-care-for-caregivers-of-mental-health-patients/
- *Seasonal Affective Disorder - National Institute of Mental Health* https://www.nimh.nih.gov/health/publications/seasonal-affective-disorder
- *Guide to Starting a Support Group* https://iocdf.org/ocd-finding-help/supportgroups/how-to-start-a-support-group/
- *An Update of Peer Support/Peer Provided Services ...* https://www.ncbi.nlm.nih.gov/pmc/articles/PMC8855026/
- *Effective use of social media platforms for promotion of mental health awareness* https://www.ncbi.nlm.nih.gov/pmc/articles/PMC7325786/
- *Seasonal Affective Disorder (SAD)* https://askjan.org/disabilities/Seasonal-Affective-Disorder-SAD.cfm
- *Prevalence of Seasonal Affective Disorder at four latitudes* https://www.researchgate.net/publication/20830480_Prevalence_of_Seasonal_Affective_Disorder_at_four_latitudes
- *Ritual, Seasonality and Affective Disorders* https://www.jstor.org/stable/3803796
- *Yoga for Depression: 9 Poses to Try* https://psychcentral.com/depression/yoga-for-depression
- *Acupuncture for Depression: A Systematic Review and Meta-Analysis* https://www.ncbi.nlm.nih.gov/pmc/articles/PMC6722678/
- *Role of Art Therapy in the Promotion of Mental Health* https://www.ncbi.nlm.nih.gov/pmc/articles/PMC9472646/
- *Green Light Therapy For Depression (Research, Best Lights ...* https://optoceutics.com/green-light-therapy-treatment-device-for-depression-mood-disorder-sad/

- *Seasonal Affective Disorder* https://www.nimh.nih.gov/health/publications/seasonal-affective-disorder
- *Seasonal Affective Disorder: "I just wanted to hibernate"* https://www.rethink.org/news-and-stories/blogs/2020/01/seasonal-affective-disorder-i-just-wanted-to-hibernate/
- *Bright Light Therapy: Seasonal Affective Disorder and ...* https://www.ncbi.nlm.nih.gov/pmc/articles/PMC6746555/
- *79 Resources for Managing Seasonal Affective Disorder* https://www.publichealthdegrees.org/resources/79-resources-managing-seasonal-affective-disorder/

Printed in Great Britain
by Amazon

53344169R00086